HEALING
AUTO IMMUNE
CONDITIONS

The detailed notes pertaining to this book are available on the HarperCollins *Publishers* India website. Scan this QR code to access the same.

HEALING AUTO IMMUNE CONDITIONS

The Holistic 6-STEP PROGRAMME to Beat Your Disease

RACHNA CHHACHHI

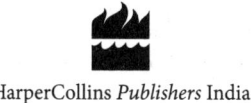

HarperCollins *Publishers* India

First published in India by HarperCollins *Publishers* 2025
Building No. 10, Tower A, 4th Floor, DLF Cyber City,
DLF Phase II, Gurugram—122002
www.harpercollins.co.in

2 4 6 8 10 9 7 5 3 1

Copyright © Rachna Chhachhi 2025

P-ISBN: 978-93-6569-519-9
E-ISBN: 978-93-6569-013-2

The views and opinions expressed in this book are the author's own
and the facts are as reported by her, and the publishers
are not in any way liable for the same.

Rachna Chhachhi asserts the moral right
to be identified as the author of this work.

All rights reserved. No part of this publication may be reproduced,
stored in a retrieval system, or transmitted, in any form or by
any means, electronic, mechanical, photocopying, recording or
otherwise, without the prior permission of the publishers.

Typeset in 11/14 Adobe Garamond Pro at
HarperCollins *Publishers* India

Printed and bound at
Replika Press Pvt. Ltd.

This book is produced from independently certified FSC® paper
to ensure responsible forest management.

Disclaimer

The contents of this book are for informational purposes only and do not substitute professional medical advice. This book should not be used to treat or diagnose any medical condition. Please consult your physician before making changes to your regular diet, or treatment. The appropriate nutrient values and allergen potential of each food source may vary for each individual. The information provided via the book is intended to be used as a guide only. All efforts have been made to present accurate and reliable information. However, the Publisher and the author do not guarantee any specific outcomes and disclaim all liability from the use or application of the contents of this book by the readers.

Vimi beat crippling multiple sclerosis with the six steps. From a prognosis of being wheelchair-bound, she now leads a full life.

Camellia, Farah and Ayse not only healed themselves from rheumatoid arthritis (RA), but also joined the autoimmune community to help others heal.

Devanshi Mago recovered from lupus nephritis after two relapses and now manages the family business at twenty-six.

Rohit Patwari thought he could never leave his home again due to his rare autoimmune condition, focal segmental glomerulosclerosis (FSGS), but today he travels internationally.

Dr Sredevi discovered lifestyle medicine after her RA treatment with me and became a lifestyle medicine healer herself.

Michel LaVire overcame depression and inflamed joints caused by RA and now helps others with chronic pain and autoimmune diseases.

Jayshree Gupta could restart her business venture, which she had abandoned due to health issues, after healing from ankylosing spondylitis (AS) and Hashimoto's.

These, and so many others, are the journeys of those who followed the path in this book, making it the voice of those who have suffered and healed from different types of autoimmune diseases. I call them 'warriors'. I too am a warrior.

We warriors want to be heard and seen in our struggles to cope with incurable conditions.

This book is dedicated to every autoimmune warrior who has been told that they're lazy, ungrateful and made to feel worthless.

We are worthy.

CONTENTS

Prologue ... ix

Part 1

1. I am a rheumatoid arthritis warrior ... 3
2. Finding others ... 19

Part 2

3. The causes are the cure ... 29
4. An immunologist's perspective ... 44
5. The six steps ... 46
6. Before you begin ... 54
7. Physical nutrition ... 57
8. Emotional nutrition ... 72
9. Music for pranayama ... 79
10. Gut repair ... 81
11. Movement ... 87
12. Talk therapy ... 106

Part 3

13. Phase 1—day zero to thirty	113
14. Phase 2—day thirty-one to ninety	126
15. Phase 3—after ninety days	136
16. Your new normal	142
17. My normal	146

Part 4

18. Feeling normal	153
19. Working with your doctor	159
20. Weird things for self-healing	162
21. Coping techniques for caregivers	167
22. Coping techniques for the warrior	172
23. Dousing flare-ups	175
24. Moving forward	178

Part 5

25. Days like this	183
100 Recipes	**189**

Gratitude	277
Notes	279
Further Reading	281
About the author	283

PROLOGUE

If I hadn't been bedridden in 2006 with joints that had been clinically deformed, I would have still been working as a gross-body[1] person in the corporate sector. Rheumatoid arthritis not only changed my life, but also made me get in touch with my own consciousness. It made me realize that what I was doing till then had no meaning and my pain and suffering had a higher purpose—to help others. My loved ones may not agree with this thinking because of the extreme suffering they witnessed and also had to go through when they saw me in that state. But they do agree that I am not the same person that I was in 2006. And that is because it's in times like these that you get perspective. You understand that what you may consider important today may not matter in three or five years.

Read this book if you are an autoimmune warrior, a caregiver to a warrior or someone on the autoimmune spectrum. Many people, especially women, don't even realize that they're on the spectrum. Low immunity, frequent coughs and colds, the flu, bronchial asthma, eczema, skin allergies, endometriosis, PCOS (polycystic ovary syndrome), poor gut health and high levels of stress combined with high emotional sensitivity are some of the triggers for an autoimmune condition. Being a woman increases your risk of this disease.[2]

An autoimmune disease is unlike any other disease. It can devastate a person's mind, body and soul. Along with the debilitating pain, brain fog, dry eyes, dry mouth and deformities, we have to live with the fact that it is incurable. Toxic medications such as chemotherapy drugs, immunosuppressants and steroids are pumped into us. They give us very little relief from the symptoms but have a highly negative impact on our gut, emotions and mental health.

Don't think of someone with an autoimmune disease as if they're lazy or incompetent. Inside that struggling body is a mind crying for help and asking you to be compassionate. Be kind. Kindness—without the pity—is all they need.

PART 1

When you try to find it, a path appears.

1

I AM A RHEUMATOID ARTHRITIS WARRIOR

Devastating. Debilitating. Excruciating. Anguished. Upsetting. Frustrating. Harrowing. Agonizing. Incurable. Impossible. Unbearable.

These were some of the words that popped up when I researched my condition. After my diagnosis in 2006, the road ahead seemed long and unforgiving at first. I had brain fog. I had pain. I was feverish. I was dull. I had dry eyes and a dry mouth. And I had to find a way to do research and collect data to heal myself in that state of mind and body. Every autoimmune warrior will understand the symptoms. Medicines don't help, assurances don't work, food doesn't bring relief, quick-fix remedies don't alleviate the pain. So, I quit the medications in 2008 to find another path.

Seventeen years later, here I am—standing, thriving, healing. Many of my orthopaedic friends ask me how I am walking because I am not 'supposed' to have any movement or mobility.

What did I do that worked?

In this book, I will share my journey of healing to help you and the entire autoimmune community understand that there is a ray of hope for us.

MY STORY

In 2006, I was diagnosed with RA. I was told by my rheumatologist that I would be deformed and bedridden if I didn't take the prescribed medications. The side effects of the medications included brain fog, hair loss, dry eyes and dry mouth. However, despite the doctor's assurances, my deformities began while on medications, specifically methotrexate. My knees, ankles and wrists were all destroyed as per my X-ray and MRI scans. Life was unbearable.

Rheumatoid arthritis is an autoimmune condition. The immune system mistakenly attacks the small joints, the synovial joints and finally all vital organs. It's a systemic disease that causes inflammation and pain in the joints, eventually leading to loss of functionality of the joint, and deformities. RA varies in severity, ranging from mild inflammation in a few small joints to symmetric inflammation in multiple joints, mainly in the hands and feet. It can happen to young people, even to children under ten. Women are twice as likely to get RA than men. According to World Health Organization (WHO) statistics, approximately 1 per cent of the population has it. There is no cure in medical science.[1]

In 2006, I was a vice president of business development at GE Money, then a Fortune 50 company. I was globetrotting and had just won the company's highest global award. My life was amazing—I had a loving husband and a beautiful daughter. I ate healthy—fruits and greens—and exercised. I was the epitome of good health.

And just like that, with the snap of a finger, a diagnosis destroyed my perfect life.

I was diagnosed quickly, unlike many of the patients whom I later treated. It took up to a year or more for some of them to receive their RA diagnosis. I went to an orthopaedic doctor who immediately referred me to a rheumatologist. Of course, I was in denial and decided to try alternative treatment instead. I had thought, *I eat healthy, I can beat this. Maybe homeopathy will work.* So, I went to a homeopath and tried her medications. She was a wonderful lady with an amazing reputation for healing. But two months later, I didn't see any results.

Then, I turned to Ayurveda. *I can still beat it without being deformed,* I thought. In Ayurveda, RA is called *Aamavata*—and just like in conventional medicine, it is considered to be an incurable condition.[2] However, I could not find any Ayurvedic doctor who could help me get better. The Ayurvedic treatments I tried made my pain worse. It was only years later when I did my MA and PhD in yoga that I realized that a large part of what I had done to heal myself overlapped with Ayurvedic treatments. But no Ayurvedic doctor I met implemented this holistic view back in 2006.

Even today, I have found that the understanding of clinical research on how to heal RA is lacking in both Ayurvedic and conventional medicine. In this book, I present the holistic treatment that has worked for me and thousands of patients across twenty-seven countries with a high clinical impact and a better quality of life outcome. Only Ayurvedic treatment can't be the cure and all studies only point to 'symptomatic relief'. That is simply because they don't focus on the emotional triggers. I tried what was available to me at the time I was trying to heal myself. I tried the fourteen-day *Panchakarma* treatment that is specifically for RA. However, my pain levels increased. I knew I had to turn to medical science.

I went to a rheumatologist, who put me on medications to manage the pain and inflammation. The medications prescribed to manage this condition—as well as other autoimmune conditions—are chemotherapy drugs such as methotrexate along with immunosuppressants and steroids, all of which damage the liver and kidneys. Every two months a blood test is required to gauge if the prescribed drugs are damaging our bodies—basically, to ensure they aren't slowly killing us.

Among the side effects are bleeding gums, swollen hands, fever, anaphylaxis, loss of appetite, nausea, headaches, diarrhoea, fatigue and drowsiness.[3] If these side effects are seen, the dosage is reduced or adjusted. If the reports are okay, the slow poisoning continues. The drugs also cause muscle wasting and suppressed haemoglobin. I lost weight and my haemoglobin dipped to 7. The normal level is above 12. If haemoglobin levels drop below 8, most doctors prescribe a blood transfusion.[4]

A distant relative who is also a doctor looked at my fragile arms, the medical patch on my inner elbow and my scanty and brittle hair and said, 'You look like a druggie.' It was not something I was expecting to hear from a family member, especially one who is a doctor. But that description gave me a realistic picture of what my quality of life was like at the time. I always remained in a daze because of the brain fog and fatigue, and I was in pain and had a limp despite the drugs.

Pretty quickly, the deformities began. My right knee swelled to the size of a football and my right wrist to that of a tennis ball. My left ankle and right foot became black due to poor circulation in my small blood vessels and my right ring finger and my right elbow were deformed for life. It was a challenge to move, let alone walk. Lifting a bottle of water became impossible. I couldn't bear to look at myself in the mirror.

I slipped into depression. The thirty-six hours of labour with my daughter seemed like a cakewalk in comparison to the pain

I was going through with this disease. And I was getting the best medical treatment. I joked that now I would qualify for a disabled person discount if we bought a car. But underneath that humour, a bitter person was emerging.

I had an extremely flourishing career, but suddenly it wasn't the same. I still had my job because my manager was a compassionate, wonderful person who believed in my potential. But then one day he left the company and one of my colleagues was promoted to manager. On a scale of 1 to 10, the new manager had an empathy score of -100. The office gossip told me that he had been aiming for the award that I eventually beat him to, so it was payback time. I needed to go for hour-long physiotherapy sessions three afternoons a week. Each time I left for a session, the new manager made it a point to be difficult in front of others, making me feel like I was worthless.

Slowly, everything I had been proud of was being taken away from me because of this disease. I took pride in my work and what I had achieved despite all odds. Even without a background in finance, I became successful in a global financial services company. My peers had Ivy League MBAs whereas I was a history honours graduate with a post-graduate diploma in journalism. But it was I who brought in the highest business revenue and won the top award at the company. Now I was unable to even work a full nine-to-five office day.

My self-worth was linked to my agility, flexibility and how I looked. I had been a dancer and had been trained in Kathak and Bharatanatyam. At family weddings, I usually did the choreography for Bollywood dances, but with my ankles and knees affected by the disease, dancing became a distant memory. I was also a painter and had held exhibitions of my art works, making good sales and earning appreciation via media coverage.

But now I couldn't hold a brush steady. And with my thinning hair, hoarse voice, tinnitus and bloodshot eyes that always felt like they had pebbles in them, I looked worse than a shadow of my previous self.

I began resenting everyone around me. I saw my husband, Vikram, get ready for work, and I resented his 'normal' state of health. I resented him being able to enjoy work when I couldn't. I was earning more than him for a part of our life together, but suddenly I felt worthless. I began feeling that he was spending more and more time at work—maybe because my long hours of pain and helplessness made that time seem longer. These thoughts, these feelings of helplessness and my poor self-worth pushed me further into a sea of depression, and I began to believe that I had become insignificant in his life. The one person whom I blindly loved and trusted, whose love I thought was rock solid, had betrayed me by not being there with me during my darkest hours. I now know I was being unreasonable, but I didn't have this perspective then.

We began to fight. And the fights were really ugly, loud and toxic. In hindsight, I can see his frustration at not getting through to me. I see the tears in his eyes that I never saw then. So consumed was I by my own self-pity that I was insensitive to him. In my mind, my marriage was on the rocks. I developed trust issues. One day I told him, 'This is so convenient, right? Now that I am of no use to you and have so much pain that I can't have sex with you, you go and enjoy yourself at work and be with all the women who are more attractive to you.' Till date, it breaks his heart when he remembers this statement.

At the same time, I was nurturing a lot of guilt about not being a good mother. Before my RA diagnosis, I felt that I was unfair to my daughter for leaving her behind when I was travelling for work. However, with the disease, there was a whole other level of guilt. My daughter, Aradhna, was a sensitive child. She was only nine at the time and all she wanted was time to cuddle with her Maa. When I was well, I made sure to read to her every night and rewarded her for reading a book every week. However, after my illness, my motivation to do anything for her became zero.

I began to neglect her. I could not take care of myself, how was I expected to take care of another human? Aradhna began to feel scared around me because I would go from being morose to yelling loudly out of frustration and pain in a matter of seconds. She could not hug me because her Maa felt so much pain, she was scared. She began tiptoeing around me, her eyes filled with fear, and began hiding food that I would not approve of. Aradhna was struggling with her own emotions with no help and support from me. Food became her solace.

No treatment seemed to be working. I was taking my meds and eating healthy, but I was only getting worse. And my family life was crumbling. Amidst all this, in 2007, I became pregnant. We had always wanted a second child—at least I did. However, my gynaecologist advised us that there was a high chance of the foetus being adversely affected by my medications. With my condition, looking after a baby with special needs would further worsen my health.

There are studies that support what my gynaecologist had once warned me about. 'Pregnant women with an autoimmune disease end a pregnancy in most cases due to serious health risks to themselves or the foetus—in some cases because they take arthritis drugs like methotrexate, mycophenolate mofetil or thalidomide, which cause birth defects.'[5] So I had to terminate my pregnancy. I had never had an abortion before.

The procedure isn't just going and getting the uterus cleaned up. Mental illness is found to be higher in women who have terminated pregnancies when compared to women without a history of abortion.[6]

Our hormones play a huge role in the level of pain we feel. The abortion completely set back my efforts to recover from RA and my pain increased drastically after the procedure. My mental health disintegrated. I felt nothing was worth living for. On two occasions, Vikram had to snatch a handful of sleeping pills from my hand. I felt like a burden. I could not even take care of myself. What would my daughter think of a mother who could not get herself a glass of water? Would my husband look at other women and then at me, thinking, *I could have that, but instead I have this.*

I was alive but I was not living. I felt like a zombie. I went to work, but everything was a blur. Yet even within this period, somewhere my hope persisted. I tried wax baths for my hands and feet to get relief, but it didn't work. I continued with physiotherapy, but the relief was temporary and marginal. My turning point came after I could not move my hands and wrists because they were so swollen and painful. My rheumatologist suggested steroid injections to reduce the inflammation.

In the span of an hour, thirteen injections were injected into my knuckles, wrists and one elbow. The needle went right into the bone, without anaesthesia. I yelled in pain. The reception, where my husband and daughter waited, was at the front of the hospital and the doctor's room was at the back. But they could clearly hear my screams. After we went home, I went to bed and don't remember much of the next three days. I am told that I was up and about for a bit, but I have no recollection of that.

When I finally regained my conscious mind, I sat up in bed only to find a mass of hair on my pillow. In disgust, I limped to the living room. Vikram and Aradhna were sitting there looking very worried. I whispered, 'I want a coffee.' My husband gently reminded me that I was not allowed to have coffee. A look of pure irritation and frustration crossed my face. He didn't want to argue as we'd been through too many fights that had left us drained and emotionally devastated. The coffee appeared.

Coffee wasn't allowed because it can increase pain in RA patients.[7] I observed that it increased my pain within thirty-six hours of consumption. I eventually had to quit drinking it. But that day, coffee did the trick. The second cup cleared up my brain fog and gave me the strength to seek a path ahead. The first thing I did was to limp from the living room to the kitchen and take out all the toxic medications from the medicine cabinet. I flushed them down the toilet. Extremely stupid, you will say. I agree. And now I had no way out. They weren't helping anyway.

Over the next few days, I did some reading and research. Back then there wasn't as much information available online, so to supplement my basic internet research I visited bookstores and libraries. Eventually, I came to a simple conclusion—if RA was an autoimmune condition, then there was something wrong with my immune system and I needed to fix it. Rheumatoid arthritis is an inflammatory condition, which meant that something in my life was triggering inflammation in my body. I began to devote all my efforts to try and understand what it was and how to fix it.

I read that in some clinical trials, Ayurveda and yoga had provided relief, but not a cure. However, Ayurveda had not worked for me. At that stage, I was desperate to try anything new. I searched for and found a yoga teacher. He was a young man who would gently work with my body. My joints were swollen and stiff, but he would sit patiently and gently rotate my ankles and wrists for me. After a few months, some movement began to return.

At the same time, I began focusing on anti-inflammatory nutrition via the elimination process. I was eating healthy, but something was triggering the inflammation. I tried to identify the foods that caused a spike in symptoms within a day or two of consumption and eventually found them to be sour foods, lentils and pulses. After eliminating them from my diet, I added more leafy greens and lots of extra-virgin olive oil (EVOO). I didn't know then that there was medical research proving the bone-protective qualities of EVOO.[8] I had always liked the taste of EVOO and since I had given up saturated fat, milk and milk products, I was using EVOO to flavour my salads. It seemed to make my joints feel better. I also identified bananas and citrus fruits as sources of increased pain and brain fog, so I eliminated them. For a while, the only fruit I ate was apples before adding papaya to my diet.

I grew up in a vegetarian household, but my father would sometimes bring home delicious non-vegetarian food. I enjoyed chicken but never developed a taste for mutton or fish. I ate chicken breast once a week until I turned nineteen, and then became completely vegetarian for nine years. I returned to eating chicken two years after getting married because Vikram was a hardcore meat-eater and I felt bad that he couldn't eat non-vegetarian food if we were together.

As part of the healing process, I needed more protein to reduce muscle fatigue. I had even eliminated dairy from my diet, so I added chicken breast to my daily meals. I had a salad with chicken and croutons and EVOO as the dressing for lunch and dinner every day. For weeks and months, this was all I ate apart from apples. The repetitive meals didn't bother me. Over time, I saw a lowering of fatigue levels and an increase in energy.

I didn't give up wheat at that time. My food plate was still 85 per cent plant-based with a humongous quantity of romaine lettuce, which became my elixir for gut repair and maintaining liver and kidney health for the rest of my life. Later I would discover that romaine lettuce is superior to other lettuce types as it is richer in polyphenols and folate.[9] Being an immunity-boosting vitamin, folate (folic acid) supplementation is required for all autoimmune patients.

THE COMBINATION WORKED

The combination of yoga with changes to my diet worked for me. I noticed my pain had reduced by about half even without medication. Most would say that it was a gigantic shift. But I didn't want to accept 50 per cent. I wanted all my life back. I had mourned my previous life and the loss of my unborn child. My poor quality of life had led me to experience emotional breakdowns, depression and suicidal thoughts. Now, I was done with all that. The lower levels of pain and higher energy had given me the strength to fight back. *I am not a victim*, I told myself. *I am a survivor.* I was not going to accept any half-hearted stuff.

THE MISSING LINK WAS RIGHT UNDER MY NOSE

In many of my conversations with my yoga teacher, he had asked me to increase my breathing exercises. But I could not do more than fifty counts of *anulom vilom* (alternate nostril breathing).

How do you concentrate on your breath when each cell in your body is hurting? Besides, I could not hold up my right elbow for too long but that movement was necessary to do anulom vilom. I would slump and give up.

As the nutrition and movement made me feel 50 per cent better, I was able to sit in one place for longer without feeling too stiff. One day, I was watching TV and unconsciously began practising alternate nostril breathing even though it was not my time of the day to do yoga. I was sitting on the sofa with my right elbow resting on the sofa arm and my feet up on a footstool. The position was comfortable. Before I knew it, I had done anulom vilom for twenty minutes! I was very proud of myself and wondered what had changed. Then I realized that the TV had kept my mind diverted and I was sitting comfortably, unlike my usual yoga position on the floor where everything poked me and increased my pain and discomfort. The next day, I once again made myself comfortable and to distract myself, I used music. It worked even better than the visual medium.

As early as the 1970s, the Mayo Clinic had done research that proved that alternate nostril breathing brought down inflammation levels.[10] As per research at Coventry University, music combined with a mind–body intervention such as slow breathing repairs the body at the DNA level.[11] In 2019, AIIMS in New Delhi published research on the benefits of yoga for RA patients.[12] I didn't know all this back in 2008, but I was utilizing the same methods to kickstart my healing.

Looking back, I feel the universe had my back. The deep dark hole I had dug myself into was starting to fill up with light. A staircase had appeared and I wanted to climb up and get out of that hole. I knew that each step would be painful, but

I had already seen the light. Something magical was happening. My response to stress was reducing, my pain levels were going down, my agility was increasing and my mind was becoming calmer. Eight months of the consistent combination of yoga and selective nutrition made me feel almost normal.

REMISSION

I decided to get my bloodwork done. Rheumatoid arthritis is diagnosed as per levels of anti-CCP antibodies, ESR, C-reactive protein and inflammation in CBC. In my new reports, everything was negative. I had a eureka moment. I thought I had found a cure to an incurable condition! But when I spoke to some doctors, I was told I was in remission. Remission is when your symptoms go away for a while. *Okay*, I thought, *why can't I permanently be in remission?* Could I not follow this healing lifestyle and make my symptoms go away forever?

Even years later, every time I worked extensive hours or experienced an emotionally stressful event, the pain would return. But it never reached the extreme levels of agony of when I was on medication. I could make the pain disappear within a couple of days with my combination of specialized nutrition and yoga. I continue to do that even today. This sustained practice is what keeps my inflammation levels down and keeps me agile, positive and healthy. It's a practice we all follow in some way. For example, if we've indulged on a holiday, when we come back, we try to detox in order to re-balance and make up for the indulgences.

SLOWING DOWN HASTENED MY JOURNEY

My experience was mine alone, but it was enough for me to quit my corporate career and study nutritional therapy at Oxford College. However, despite my desire to help others to get healthier, I had no experience in the field of therapy. I didn't think that I was a good listener or that my personality was naturally adaptive to being patient. I had been successful in my previous career because I had been restless, ambitious and quick at learning, adapting and implementing. Now, I had to slow down. I had to pause and be patient.

I was no longer in a high-pressure job that pushed me to be hurried all the time. I took time out in the day to ensure that I ate well, did my yoga and breathing practices and reflected on how I could become a healer. The slower pace made my mind work faster. My brain was no longer under the pressure of deadlines or being subject to extreme pain and brain fog. It was working at lightning speed. My new life had begun, one in which I would feel better and would help others. The aggressive corporate go-getter in me began to slowly disappear and be replaced by a calmer person. I was no longer in a hurry, no longer running around in a frenzy to prove myself to others. I learnt that to 'unhurry' was to heal.

When I began my career as a healer, some people saw it as a passing phase and thought that I would soon give up. I just kept my head down and got my nutritional therapy certification. I clinically healed my first patient in 2009. After that, my work spoke for itself. My gratitude demonstrated my commitment. If people doubt you but you believe in yourself, don't pay heed to them. They are judging you based on their own life experiences. Nothing can stop you if you believe in yourself and follow that up with hard work.

It's been fifteen years since I started on this second life journey. In each of those years, I study a new area of healing to help those without hope of recovery. I did 200 hours of training to become a yoga teacher, eventually getting a master's degree in the subject. Presently I'm finishing my PhD in yoga. I also became a certified cancer metastasis expert from Johns Hopkins University and was certified in malnutrition in infants and children in a programme by the WHO taskforce. After that, I completed a certificate course in Positive Psychiatry and Mental Health from the University of Sydney. Today, I run a registered non-profit organization where we have a community to support warriors.

Nutrition, yoga and breathwork have remained the backbone for me. However, it's not that I never had a relapse. Many people mistakenly think that if they're in remission, they can go back to their previous lives, before their disease was triggered. Doing that will only bring the symptoms back. Healing autoimmune conditions can be compared to losing weight. Usually, to lose weight we go on a programme where we exercise regularly and eat healthy. After losing the weight, if we go back to our previous life of stress, not exercising and consuming junk food, we will gain it back. But no doctor tells a patient who has lost weight that they're 'in remission'.

It's the same with type-2 diabetes, heart disease and autoimmune conditions. The life that gave you your condition has to be left behind and a new normal needs to be embraced and respected. For warriors, the biggest trigger for flare-ups is stress. I had three relapses in fifteen years. These were all triggered by emotionally stressful events—my mother's passing was one of them. But I recovered very quickly without medications.

In this book, I help you understand how to accept the stress in a passive manner rather than be reactive, and how to stay in remission constantly. I help you cure your autoimmune condition and follow your new normal while you have a wonderful quality of life. The question is, will you commit to this new normal? Because you can have everything if you are willing to commit to yourself.

As I write this, I am sitting in a café in Frankfurt. A couple of days later I will be in Paris. I walk, exercise, eat out, treat patients across the world, write books, I am invited as a speaker to medical conferences internationally where senior leaders and the medical community want to understand my case studies and how to be healthy. My non-profit foundation works to spread awareness about nutrition, mental health and sustainable living. Our NGO does free camps on mental health and malnutrition for autoimmune warriors, the underprivileged, organizations and security forces. I have my hands full. Anyone in my place would have fatigue, extra workload or even a relapse. But there are ways to avoid this and stay on the path and keep healing mentally and physically.

You can too. You can have everything, if you are willing to commit to yourself.

2

FINDING OTHERS

Equipped with my shiny new certification, I began my healing practice in 2009. I was excited to help autoimmune warriors because I understood their struggles. I yearned to reach out and hug them and tell them that all their broken parts would be fixed by this holistic approach. I had a diploma in nutritional therapy and my own experience of healing to build on. It was going to be easy.

But I had quit my corporate career, and I didn't have any money. So, I decided to start small by first creating a website with a contact form. I then wrote articles about my journey and published them on a couple of health websites. A health magazine, *Prevention*, published my story. While I waited, I kept doing more research. I was hoping to hear from people struggling with autoimmune conditions, so I was surprised to get more queries related to weight loss, arthritis in the fingers, increasing height and type-2 diabetes. Since I was certified to treat these cases, I accepted them.

I was surprised to find that the same methodology to reduce inflammation in the body by using nutrition and breathwork seemed to work clinically for all the other conditions that people came to me for. A strict regimen of healthy foods along with breathing exercises and yoga worked to help people clinically reverse their lifestyle diseases. But my mission was to reduce the daily suffering faced by autoimmune patients where 'generally healthy foods' don't work.

Back then, there was very little information available about autoimmune diseases, so I decided to open a physical clinic to supplement my online practice. Perhaps having a physical space people could walk into would give more patients around my geography the confidence to consult with me. To do so, I had to borrow money from dad and from Vikram—later, I paid them both back. This allowed me to pay the rent for a clinic room in a co-working space.

The decision made the difference and soon autoimmune warriors within India began contacting me, and those from other countries seemed to feel reassured that I had a physical clinic. Whether it was the sweet gentle Danielle from Cape Town, South Africa, who had RA, the beautiful and brave Preet Kamal Brar from Seattle, USA, who had irritable bowel syndrome (IBS), or Vimi Gupta from Bengaluru who had chronic multiple sclerosis (MS) for fourteen years, or parents of little children who had conditions like juvenile arthritis, Wegener's—they all got in touch with me. I documented some of these cases in my first book, *Restore*.

Danielle's case brings a ray of hope to all of us if there is early diagnosis. She was just twenty-six years old when she contacted me. She had been told by her rheumatologist that she could lead a normal life only by taking seven pills once a week. However, some research led her to understand that the rheumatologist had prescribed her cancer drugs. Danielle refused to accept that she had to endure that for the rest of her life and had faith in the holistic approach towards healing herself, and she wanted my help to safely wean herself off methotrexate.

Danielle told me that she was eager to try my treatment plan of adopting an anti-inflammatory lifestyle and eating anti-inflammatory foods. 'I am a mentally and emotionally strong individual and I believe I will be able to reverse my RA with your help,' she wrote in her contact form. I emailed her back with my methodology for online treatment that included video sessions and email support. Together, we soon identified that her triggers were emotional.

Within three months of starting treatment, I had clinically reversed Danielle's condition and her symptoms had disappeared, so much so that when she went for her next health checkup, the doctor who had diagnosed her with RA was doubtful that she ever had it! When I recently got back in touch with her, she told me that she had been healthy for years. 'It took me some time to realize that while I had initially attributed my healing to diet, it was connecting with my body through yoga that was the real catalyst,' she said. 'I was completely unaware that I had childhood trauma lodged in my body that made me ill, a common response as the mind subconsciously blocks out memories that are too painful to bear.' By learning to connect with the present moment, Danielle was able to learn how to trust her body and feel a sense of safety, which allowed her nervous system to regulate and process emotions. It released her belief systems and eliminated the disease.

CHILDHOOD TRAUMA AS A TRIGGER

A direct relationship between childhood stress and autoimmune diseases has been established, with the findings presented in the research paper 'Cumulative Childhood Stress and Autoimmune Diseases in Adults.'[1] I often see childhood trauma being the trigger, and yoga the healer in many autoimmune warriors I treat.

In my first session with a warrior who signs up for my treatment, I ask them what they feel their trigger is. At this time, they're usually not ready to acknowledge what happened in their childhood. The immediate trigger is an event three to five years before their diagnosis. Over the next few months, I explore deeper into their childhood. Sometimes the trauma isn't perceived. For example, in my case, just being made to grow up faster than normal robbed me of my childhood. When I was eleven, I remember my parents saying that I will manage everything on my own. It made me feel that even at that age I was responsible for resolving my problems on my own.

It was also perceived as my duty to resolve the conflicts my brother had with other family members. My brother is three years older than me. When he was a child, he was mischievous bordering on wicked. Slowly, his behaviour turned into destructiveness, but no one sat him down to understand why he behaved that way. I had to play peacemaker at home if anything related to him erupted into ugly fights and raised voices.

To deal with my stress, I would disappear in the backyard with my dog, read and overeat. I soon gained weight and had to endure the jibes of relatives, friends, loved ones and everyone else who thought my weight was their business. I was not pretty like my mom, nor was I intelligent like my brother—I was just a fat, dumb kid who was expected to fend for herself without any guidance. I began to exercise and eat healthy by age thirteen and had lost 20 kg by the time I turned sixteen. After we grew up, my brother and I often wondered why we were never hugged by our parents. Their affection was more verbal and infrequent because they were very busy with their work or firefighting battles with the extended family. I was still given a lot of affection by my father, but my brother experienced less of that when he was growing up. Very often I would be caught in a crossfire between two alpha males and since both of them listened to me, the dependency on me dousing the fire between two men I loved unconditionally became very high.

As an adult, I can now appreciate my mother's struggles and despair. We always had relatives from my father's side of the family visiting us, even staying with us for days on end. With the demands of family, housework and her social life, she barely got any time for herself. She lived to meet her husband's needs. It wasn't like my father made too many demands, but because, from the beginning, she had done everything for him, it became an expectation. But she was pouring from an empty cup. Towards the end, she became bitter about his demands. I think this is the scenario with most women of that generation.

At thirty-nine, my mother had a bout of RA herself. She recalled that even her grandmother had RA at a young age. In those times, the colloquial name for the sickness was *gathia*. It took her about eight months to recover. Funnily, as I write this, I'm recalling that it also took me eight months to heal. When mom was bedridden, I learnt how to cook because she couldn't, with her right hand swollen and rigid. The orthopaedic surgeon who treated her was an army doctor whose son died of complications from juvenile RA at the age of fourteen. For him, healing my mother became a personal mission—and he was successful.

Unfortunately, by the time of my diagnosis, that doctor was no more. My mother said she wished she had kept her medical documents from the time. 'All I remember is him giving me a bunch of different coloured tablets, I think they were vitamins,' she said. 'And he was giving me ibuprofen two or three times a day.' I recalled that he had asked her to rest completely, take the medicines and leave home only for physiotherapy. Slowly she began getting the movement back her in right hand with the physiotherapy, all the while having only vitamins and painkillers as medication.

My mother had received immediate medical attention after diagnosis. This was similar to Danielle, who too had recovered with immediate intervention. My mother lived to almost seventy-eight and never had an autoimmune flare-up again. My brother and I agree that her RA had been triggered by the stress in her marriage. I was lucky to have many conversations with my mom about this before she passed. She would often cry and say that she was so busy being a good wife that she forgot to be a good mother too. We became closer than we had ever been, and I found my closure for my childhood traumas in those conversations.

But those traumas did mean that my carefree childhood was stifled. I am not alone in this experience as a warrior, most of whom have a similar trigger. Vimi Gupta, who was diagnosed with MS in 2000, says that she was an emotionally sensitive child, and witnessed fights in her family as well as experienced helplessness at her father's muscular dystrophy. 'This took a toll on my mother the most,' she recalls. 'This situation hit me badly in my adolescence. The family fights and the illness really affected me. School was my refuge. It was only after college that I understood what my father was suffering from! Till today I regret that I was unable to do anything for him.'

OUR COMMUNITY HEALS US

At every autoimmune community meet, we discuss our individual journeys as a support group. Usually the most difficult thing to talk about is how warriors arrived at the diagnosis.

Our autoimmune community is now 140-warriors strong and growing. Each one of them battles different kinds of symptoms on a daily basis. During our periodic support group meetings, warriors discuss their struggles and joys.

Finding others has helped me find my purpose and stay healed myself. For an autoimmune warrior, finding a purpose to wake up every morning for is important because it makes us feel empowered to move forward. It becomes important for us to remember that there is support available for our journey, no matter where we are.

PART 2

The wonderful thing about time is that you can't squander it beforehand. The upcoming year, day and hour are all waiting for you, flawless and untarnished. You have the option to start fresh every hour.

PART 2

3

THE CAUSES ARE THE CURE

In 1964, Norman Cousins, then the editor of *The Saturday Review of Literature*, was hospitalized with an autoimmune disease called ankylosing spondylitis (AS). He documented his healing journey in his book *Anatomy of an Illness* and followed it up by publishing a research paper in *New England Journal of Medicine* to document it as clinical research. 'I made the joyous discovery that ten minutes of genuine belly laughter had an anaesthetic effect and would give me at least two hours of pain-free sleep,' he wrote in his book, adding that the hospital's most serious failure was in the area of nutrition.[1] 'It was not just the meals that were poorly balanced; what seemed inexcusable to me was the profusion of processed foods,' he writes, stating that 'a great failure of medical schools is that they pay so little attention to the science of nutrition.'[2]

Cousins theorized that if stress could worsen his condition, then positive emotions could improve it. With the approval of his doctor, he prescribed himself a nutritious diet, a regimen of humorous videos and shows and high doses of vitamin C—as pure ascorbic acid. This 'unscientific' foundation that was published as a research paper by Cousins was included in academic medical research by Dr Lee Berk, a preventive care specialist and psychoneuroimmunologist. Berk and his colleagues discovered that anticipation of 'mirthful laughter' had surprising and significant effects. 'Beta-endorphins—the family of chemicals that elevates the mood—and human growth hormone (HGH)—which helps with increasing immunity—increased by 27 per cent and 87 per cent respectively in those who anticipated watching a humorous video. There was no such increase among the control group who didn't anticipate watching the humorous film.'[3]

In another study, 'the same anticipation of mirthful laughter reduced levels of cortisol (termed the "steroid stress hormone") by 39 per cent; epinephrine (also known as adrenaline) by 70 per cent; and dopac (the major catabolite of dopamine) by 38 per cent, compared to the control group.'[4] If chronically released, these stress hormones can be detrimental to the immune system. Researchers at the University of California in Berkeley published a paper to support the anti-inflammatory properties of vitamin C in bringing down the inflammation marker C-reactive protein.[5] This biomarker of inflammation is high in autoimmune conditions.

Cousins cured his autoimmune condition, became a professor of psychiatry and biobehavioural sciences and lived to seventy-five. Laughter and vitamin C helped him lead a good life. Yet, medical science still claims to look for a cure.

Jayshree Gupta was forty years old when she came to me with a positive HLA-B27, the clinical marker for AS. She had pain in her lower back and knees, stiffness in her shoulders, headaches, strained eyes and digestive issues like constipation. It took three years just to get diagnosed. 'I was just put on psychiatric medicines without any information on what I had,' says Jayshree, who was prescribed pills for depression, antipsychotics and epilepsy. She was also on homeopathy. Even though her HLA-B27 was positive, she was treated only for depression, never for AS.

Jayshree had chronic fatigue and low iron levels. With three antidepressants a day, her body was lethargic. She was 5 feet tall but weighed 69 kg, so her petite frame was overwhelmed and that increased her pain levels further. 'Being unwell for a long time and figuring out what to do next was challenging,' she says. Chronic stress was her trigger for severe symptoms, but it took her a long time to believe that holistic treatment would work. Still, she tried it since no other treatment had. 'It was the last hope for me,' she says, 'but after a few months of dedication, the results began to show and now a new chapter of my life has begun.'

I diagnosed Hashimoto's disease along with AS, as her thyroid antibodies were high and iron levels low, and we began treatment. Within three months, Jayshree's levels came crashing down. She lost 14 kg which reduced the pressure on her spine, and her other test results all returned to normal. Her Hashimoto's markers like microsomal TPO crashed from 257.7 to 45.8, back in range, anti-thyroglobulin antibody went down from 116.8 to 15.95. 'Before I began working with Rachna, I was really struggling with severe headaches, continuous vomiting, constipation, fatigue, joint pains, brain fog, and wanted to end my life,' reveals Jayshree. 'Today I want to start a new life. Once you adapt to this programme, it's not an effort to carry forward.' Jayshree had given up her unique business of custom-fit lingerie because she had no energy. But after her treatment, she could restart her business and it's now doing very well. She is also an active member of our autoimmune community support group and regularly takes part in non-profit events run by my foundation.

The struggles that Jayshree and so many others in similar situations face in just getting up in the morning, their emotional meltdowns and digestive issues—all of these begin disappearing when you remain consistent with a structured self-nurturing programme. That is how you make yourself healthy again. Once you are healthy and physically and mentally agile, going back to the earlier lifestyle that gave you suffering and trauma seems destructive.

There are over eighty autoimmune conditions.[6] Doctors aren't sure why we get autoimmune diseases or why women are impacted more than men. Research also suggests that higher levels of hormones in women, especially during the childbearing years, can make women more susceptible.[7] However, prepuberty children get autoimmune conditions too. I have personally treated nine-year-olds (both boys and girls).

Theses is no 'one-size-fits-all' treatment of anti-inflammatory foods, yogic exercises and breathing. We have to dive into the root cause of each individual's illness to repair their immune system and gut. If other treatments didn't work for you, it is because none of the root causes were addressed. I'll explain these root causes below.

1. OVERREACTIVE IMMUNE SYSTEM

Our immune system is complex and highly intelligent. Its mission is simple: to seek and kill invaders. If someone is born with a severely defective immune system, they're at risk of death from infections caused by various pathogens. If someone is immuno-deficit, the lack of even a single enzyme can result in the build-up of toxic waste inside immune cells, killing healthy cells and devastating the immune system.[8]

We all have innate immunity and adaptive immunity. The body's innate immunity is its initial defence against germs entering the body. The immune system reacts uniformly to all germs and foreign substances, earning it the nickname 'nonspecific' immune system. It operates swiftly, as seen when it identifies and eliminates bacteria that enter through a wound in just a few hours. But its ability to prevent the spread of germs is somewhat limited.[9]

If the innate immune system can't destroy germs, the adaptive immune system takes over. It targets the specific type of germ causing the infection, but it needs to identify the germ first. This makes its response slower than the innate immune system, but more precise. The adaptive immune system can also 'remember' germs, so it can respond quickly when it encounters a known germ again.

This immune system memory is also the reason why there are some infections you can get only once in your life, because afterwards your body becomes 'immune' to it. After the first encounter with a germ, the adaptive immune system may require a few days to respond. However, upon subsequent exposure, the body can react more quickly. As a result, the second infection is typically either unnoticeable or less severe. The adaptive immune system is made up of:

- T-lymphocytes
- B-lymphocytes
- Antibodies

The above three have a function in the diagnosis and blood biochemistry of autoimmune diseases. Imbalance or emotional reactivity can trigger an autoimmune condition. One of the main characteristics of autoimmune diseases is the breakdown of B-cell tolerance, which leads to an immune response against the body's own tissues, and triggers overproduction of autoantibodies.[10]

Simply put, the adaptive immune system becomes imbalanced and overreactive. Most autoimmune disorders result from either an excessive immune response or an 'autoimmune attack'.

A key part of the immune system's role is to single out the invaders from the body's own cells. When it fails to do so, it triggers an autoimmune disease. A warrior's immune system has the following traits:

- overreaction
- inflammation
- self-attack
- self-invasion
- toxins/pathogens
  a. virus
  b. fungus
  c. bacterium

And in these five points lies the cure. Because when each one of these is addressed, the immune system will work for us and not against us.

A faulty emotional immunity jams physical immunity

Every autoimmune warrior that I have treated, including myself, has an emotionally sensitive personality. We are emotional to the extent of causing inadvertent self-damage. This damage may not be at a physical level. Overthinking, overreacting to our external environment and putting ourselves down are the common traits I see and have personally experienced. I had to work hard to correct them in myself. Self-attack, being judgemental of oneself, self-doubt—all trigger inflammatory responses.

Emotionally vulnerable people are also easier targets for viruses, fungi and bacteria. The immune and emotional responses have been found to have similarities and overlaps in research conducted over the past few decades. The term 'emotional immunity' stems from this belief. Most living beings use physical and emotional immunity to adjust to their changing external environment. Both systems can be protective for the body if kept in control but detrimental when they're in turmoil.[11]

I'm not saying that everyone who has emotional over-reactivity will get an autoimmune condition. However, every autoimmune patient that I have treated has had emotional triggers and over-reactivity to past turmoil. Chronic stress can trigger the emotional immunity imbalance. Physical and emotional immunity develop simultaneously, so when one becomes defective, the other often follows suit. Both need to be healthy to protect us.

Childhood trauma becomes part of our emotional vulnerability. This was true for Ayse Turkmen, forty-four, who lives in Cyprus. After she contacted me for help with her RA, I learnt that her parents divorced about a year before her RA started. She had been in high school then. 'I had to take care of my younger brother, cook, clean our home and iron my father's work clothes while also keeping up my studies,' she recalls. 'My duties were too much, but I felt that I had to be strong and take care of my father and brother.' Not everyone in Ayse's situation would have had a trigger for an autoimmune disease. However, the overactive emotional immunity triggered her overthinking and she felt overwhelmed with her circumstances. This reactivity is the common thread among all warriors. It triggers the disease even in situations where other people with less emotional reactivity would not get it.

In the above scenario, pathogens weaken the system and gut even more when a person's physical and emotional immunity are unhealthy. The digestive system starts becoming weak and permeable. An emotionally sensitive person will have a weaker gut. In patients with IBS or indigestion, there is a distinct brain-to-gut pathway in which psychological symptoms begin first, and the disease begins with gut symptoms.[12]

'My father was in the US while my mother was in India taking care of my paternal grandmother,' recalls Preet Kamal Brar, a forty-five-year-old from Seattle. 'So, I was sent away to boarding school. My parents loved me a lot, but I think being away from home and not getting that care and nurturing environment affected me.' Brar developed ulcerative colitis. She had to get an ileostomy[13] and now has an ostomy bag.[14]

For many warriors, childhood trauma is a trigger because we have been holding it in for just too long.

2. GENES

Genes are our building blocks for growth and development. They influence many features, including our looks, the colour of our hair and eyes and our height. Scientists have been investigating the genetic connection of autoimmune diseases due to the higher occurrence of these conditions within the same family and in certain populations.[15]

Familial predisposition has also been identified within autoimmune diseases, particularly in RA and systemic lupus erythematosus (SLE).[16] Interestingly, it's not always the same disease. A woman whose mother has RA may develop SLE. Scientific evidence demonstrates that environmental and lifestyle factors influence epigenetic mechanisms such as DNA methylation,[17] histone modifications[18] and microRNA expression.[19] And microRNAs can regulate the production of cytokines (a type of protein made by immune and non-immune cells that impacts the immune system), which play a pivotal role in the initiation of autoimmune diseases. Understanding the role of genetics in autoimmunity can help us prevent disease triggers and customize treatments for autoimmune diseases in the future.

But often, we can't control how our children face or respond to stress in their lives. Three generations of women in my family had RA, and my daughter has fibromyalgia. Aradhna was just eighteen when she was diagnosed. 'When I was first diagnosed with fibromyalgia,' she recalls, 'I experienced mixed emotions because of how much the pain and fatigue had already impacted my moods and my movement. I was apprehensive of what it would do to my quality of life.'

Aradhna, now twenty-seven, remembers the frustration of having to give up her diploma course in design and photography just a few months before completion—which she was passionate about. 'It made my pain worse,' she says. 'I began questioning my future goals and was confused about what I would tell my friends and whether they would understand.' But none of this overwhelmed her as much as she thought it would, because she could always talk to her parents about her doubts. 'They are my secure space,' she says, 'and that feeling is what got me through.'

Even at eighteen, Aradhna was already convinced about the value of consistency and having a routine. She knew the importance of community and speaking to your loved ones in a safe space. She slowed down, rested and practised pranayama. 'I am still continuously surprised by how much these practices can help pain and mental health,' she says. Subsequently, Aradhna became a certified holistic nutrition expert, yin yoga teacher and a women's hormones specialist. 'My biggest learning from my mother, my own healing and this condition is that even when you feel down and question life, it's important to remember that you *will* get through it.'

In Aradhna's case, her genetic predisposition was combined with the childhood trauma of seeing her mother suffer. Many mother-daughter warriors with different autoimmune conditions come to me for treatment. We have a clear predisposition to an autoimmune condition because of our genetic makeup. What we need to understand is that this genetic response can be changed by lifestyle modifications. This has also been proven by the field of epigenetics.

Epigenetics is a field of research where we modify gene behaviour without altering the DNA sequence. By following specialized nutrition, reducing the response to stress and changing the immune system response from attacking or triggering the disease, to protecting the gene response, epigenetics changes gene reactivity from active to passive.[17] The same genes that are supposed to trigger our disease start becoming dormant because of the epigenetic changes from lifestyle modifications.

Dubai-based Rishika Malhotra, forty-one, came to me with lichen planopilaris and scarring alopecia. 'My mother has RA and she has overcome a lot of her pain with your treatment,' she recalls. Rishika's son, who had previously been diagnosed with lichen planus, is also better. 'Mostly when the doctor recommended eight months of oral steroids, twelve months of topical steroids and other meds and steroids shots in my scalp, is when Rachna came to mind and I reached out,' she laughs and says. Rishika is doing well today, and her alopecia is in remission.

3. LEAKY GUT

When the microbial balance in your gut is balanced, your body functions optimally. But when there is imbalance due to chronic stress, chronic constipation, exposure to environmental toxins such as pesticides, poor nutrition, pathogens or taking frequent antibiotics that wipe out a lot those microbes—the 'bad' bacteria cut holes in the gut's fence and some of them, along with food particles and toxins, leak into the bloodstream, and that's how intestinal permeability begins.[20] So when your immune system sees organisms where they don't belong, it attacks them, causing irritation and inflammation.

Those with an autoimmune condition have increased intestinal permeability. This means that their gut lets more than water and nutrients through. They 'leak' because the barriers that protect the gut lining get broken down. Studies have shown that people with leaky guts let larger molecules through, some of which could be potentially toxic.[21] Immunoglobulin-A (IgA), an immune marker, is one of the barriers that stops toxins from entering the gut. IgA protects the gut mucosal tissues from this bad bacteria invasion to maintain immune homeostasis within the gut flora. But when this fence is broken, IgA levels rise to protect the person.

The layers of the gut provide defence based on innate and acquired immunity cells by secreting IgA, cytokines, chemokines (proteins responsible for cell migration) and mast cell proteases (cells that regulate immune response). There are also endocrine and secretion mechanisms mediated by the enteric nervous system (ENS), which regulate immune response and detect nutrients. These help with the secretion of toxins.

Serotonin is an important transmitter produced in the gut. It regulates messaging between neurons present in the gut and the brain and affects sleep, mood and memory. Ninety per cent of serotonin is produced in the gut. Serotonin is found in cells along the gastrointestinal tract and is absorbed by blood platelets. Gut serotonin, or circulating serotonin, is also responsible for the regulation of blood flow, body temperature and digestion.

Low levels of serotonin can result in any number of seemingly unrelated symptoms, including fatigue, shortness of breath, neurologic symptoms, joint pain, blood clots, heart palpitation and digestive problems. Studies suggest that nutrients, prebiotics and even plant extracts improve gut-barrier function and increase serotonin.[22] Tryptophan, the precursor to serotonin, is found in eggs, fish and leafy green vegetables.[23] This demonstrates how important the right nutrition is for the production of serotonin in the gut, which regulates your moods, and is yet another example of how the mind and body are connected.

Disruption of this microbial balance causes leaky gut syndrome and inhibits vagus nerve signals. Our vagus nerve is our longest nerve in the autonomic nervous system, and has parasympathetic control of numerous organs—including the lungs, heart and diaphragm. A poor signal between the gut and the brain contributes to fatigue, gut issues and emotional turbulence. In Ayurveda, the connection between the vagus nerve and *vata dosha* has been established via clinical research and literature.[24] The vagus nerve is a modulator of the brain–gut axis in mental and inflammatory disorders.[25]

When we realize that stress in the gut and mind communicate with each other via the vagus nerve, we understand that when one gets better, so does the other. However, when rheumatologists prescribe toxic medications, they ravage the already compromised gut and disrupt its signals to the brain. This creates a spiral of anxiety because the vagus nerve is passing on the stress message triggered by immune suppressants, steroids and chemotherapy drugs. It destroys the gut flora further and the vagus nerve sends this distress signal from the gut to the brain and vice versa. The vicious cycle continues, leading to an overwhelming amount of chronic fatigue and poor gut health.

4. ADRENAL INSUFFICIENCY

Extreme and debilitating fatigue is the most common symptom among autoimmune warriors.[26] Approximately 98 per cent of those suffering from an autoimmune condition report that they suffer from fatigue. Fatigue can cause dramatic impairments in mood, diminish social and community interactions, lead to an inability to perform routine daily activities and limit physical activity and work. This fatigue can be cruel to the quality of life and well-being of the warrior, and also impact them financially.

Prolonged periods of exhaustion result in an inability to perform even simple daily activities that may seem normal to people without autoimmune conditions. Evidence points to several biological functions that trigger fatigue, including oxygen and nutrient supply, metabolism, mood, motivation and daytime sleepiness. This cognitive fatigue or brain fog reduces alertness, mental acclimatization and performance during simple every day tasks, sparking feelings of being overwhelmed very quickly.

Autoimmune diseases including IBS, MS and RA have a high association with anxiety, depression and pain, all of which induce this fatigue. Often, the outer layer of the adrenal glands—known as the 'cortex'—can't make enough hormones. This is a condition called 'primary adrenal insufficiency'.[27] This adrenal insufficiency can trigger adrenal fatigue because hormones like cortisol, DHEA, aldosterone, adrenaline and noradrenaline that reverse this fatigue are not being produced properly. It's common to see this in autoimmune warriors.

5. STRESS

Stress is everywhere and we all experience it. But when you have poor physical and emotional immunity, a poor gut and adrenal insufficiency that causes chronic fatigue, the presence of emotionally traumatic stress can trigger an autoimmune condition. According to research, it's the stress-triggered neuroendocrine hormones that ultimately lead to immune dysregulation. This results in an autoimmune disease because it alters or amplifies cytokine production.[28] Stress then becomes the proverbial last straw that triggers the disease.

Incorporating stress management and behavioural interventions can help prevent stress-related immune imbalances. It's important to discuss different stress reactions with patients with autoimmune conditions to identify potential trigger factors. But in mainstream medical science, possible triggers for the autoimmune condition are never discussed when a patient goes to the rheumatologist.

Though stress never goes away, how we react to the stress can be changed. This change of mindset is intertwined in my holistic treatment. Stress can be behind all the other root causes of autoimmune disease. Emotional immunity becomes imbalanced, and a leaky gut can be triggered due to stress. So, to heal the warrior, a change of response to stress is the primary focus.

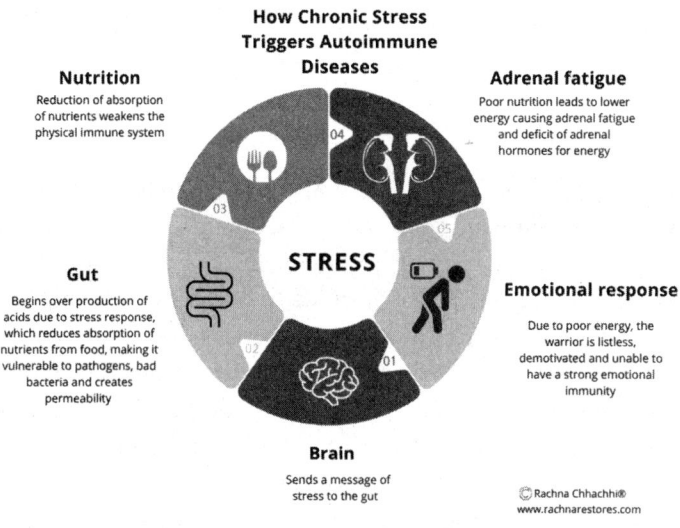

4

AN IMMUNOLOGIST'S PERSPECTIVE

I met Dr Taruna Madan Gupta when she got in touch with me about her husband's psoriasis. Dr Gupta is an immunologist who serves as the head of development research at the Indian Council of Medical Research (ICMR). She shares not only her journey of supporting her spouse through his autoimmune journey, but also provides her scientific perspective about autoimmune conditions. 'As an immunologist, I understand what is going on in my husband's body and mind,' she says, 'yet there are times when I feel completely helpless.' Everyone who has been a caregiver for a warrior has experienced this helplessness.

Dr Gupta points to stress being the main cause of autoimmune disease. 'Stress increases the level of inflammation,' she says. 'Inflammation is good for things such as tissue repair, angiogenesis and the formation of new blood vessels. But when it becomes chronic, it's resistive. The immune cells become fatigued, unable to perform their functions efficiently—not unlike our own behaviour under stress.' Stress continuously fuels pain, stiffness and skin issues or damages parts of the body attacked by our immune system. But when we actively start reducing inflammation with physical and emotional nutrition, there is a scientifically measurable outcome that shows the ability of the human body and mind to repair itself by just eating right and reducing stress levels.

'So let us not only nourish ourselves with what is on our plate but also do the same for our minds and souls so that we can reduce the flare-ups and pain,' says Dr Gupta. She talks about the struggles her husband, Sanjeev, has had to endure with his skin condition, which has sometimes led to people being unwilling to even shake his hand. 'What does medical science do?' she asks. 'It doesn't offer a cure except for management and control for a specific amount of time, beyond which the drugs don't work. Controlling your inflammation levels, stress and antibodies is the key. You can achieve this by changing your response to stress.'

Dr Gupta explains how nutrition impacts us at our DNA level. 'Telomeres are segments of the chromosomes at the end of our DNA. They shorten with age and lengthen with a good lifestyle,' she elaborates. 'Nutritionally superior lifestyles have clinically shown to lengthen our telomeres, which means we *can* repair our DNA. What you eat is definitely important, but how you eat and how you respond to the thoughts in your mind are also equally important,' Dr Gupta points out. 'Holistic treatment has clinically proven to show epigenetic changes in the body and reduce disease activity.'

She believes that we should taper off medicines once a patient is showing signs of remission. The protocols for this process must be defined and backed by clinical trials. One needs to strengthen nutrition to reduce the effect of harsh drugs. Medicines and nutrition together will help you and your family live a good life and provide a complete cure for the disease. 'If as a scientist I felt helpless about my husband's psoriasis, imagine how suffering families out there feel,' concludes Dr Gupta. 'They need help to implement this knowledge to get a better life.'

5
THE SIX STEPS

Devanshi Mago was twenty years old when her father, Sanjay, emailed me about her condition. Devanshi had been suffering from lupus for nine years by then. She doesn't remember any triggers when she was first diagnosed. However, when she relapsed, she suffered from severe joint pain. At the time of relapse, she was under a lot of stress as she was studying to get into medical school and her grandmother had passed away. The medicines affected her kidneys, and a renal biopsy diagnosed her with lupus nephritis class 4.

I had treated lupus successfully before but had experienced mixed results with lupus nephritis till then. I was frank with Sanjay about this. Sanjay was overwhelmed and grateful. The very fact that I had displayed transparency and a clear intention of helping Devanshi helped them decide to proceed further. And so, we began the treatment. Devanshi was very annoyed with the dietary restrictions at first. 'I was always cranky and angry,' she recalls. 'I would fight with my family because the *chatkara* (sour and spicy) taste that I loved was gone.' But when she started to feel her morning stiffness go away, she began to accept this treatment. 'The supplements and oil capsules worked wonders on me,' she says. 'I think it started to have a positive impact in only three weeks, but I was too annoyed at being denied my *chatkara* food to acknowledge the positive impact of the treatment.' Her family began eating the same food prescribed to her to support her in her journey, and make sure she didn't feel alone.

'I used to have severe joint pains especially in winter and would not be able to get out of bed,' says Devanshi, 'but now I don't have any joint pains even though I am not as strict with my diet and exercise. I never believed in the holistic nutrition autoimmune protocol but honestly it worked miraculously for me.' Devanshi completed her post-graduate studies in biochemistry. She is twenty-six now and runs the family business and lives a full life.

AUTOIMMUNE TREATMENT PROTOCOL

My autoimmune treatment protocol, trademarked as the RachnaRestores Protocol®, has steps for healing that can lead one to a quality of life higher than what is possible through medication. Of course, medicines are necessary to provide stopgap relief or douse emergency situations, which is the primary function of medical science. However, autoimmune diseases have no cure and the methods to alleviate symptoms are not well understood. But when we systematically approach the causes of the disease, the immune system flourishes.

This approach helps you avoid emergencies and provides relief in a matter of just a few weeks, as many of the warriors I have treated and those interviewed for this book have shared. This isn't an overnight process but a vertical line of healing that takes the autoimmune warrior from a state of demotivation to one of positivity and hope for the future. As was the case with Devanshi and many other warriors, beginning the journey is difficult—but when your symptoms begin to reduce, reports get better, your motivation to beat the disease increases.

Every autoimmune patient struggles daily with symptoms that stop them from living a normal life. In most cases, there is little motivation to do more because doctors have already declared them incurable. The patient has accepted that they will only get worse and that they have to accept the toxic side effects of medications. When someone is in a state of mind where hopelessness is the overriding emotion, just getting them to take the first step becomes difficult. Hence, we have to help them experience small wins.

My treatment takes a year for a warrior to cement the physical and emotional equilibrium in their immunity. The steps are sequential and should be followed in the order that they have been listed. The end result is reduction in overreactivity of the immune system at an emotional level as well as a body cleansed of pathogens. However, not following the sequence correctly can mess up the signalling for the central nervous system and parasympathetic nervous system, causing fatigue and flare-ups. Many warriors have tried to take shortcuts by changing or merging the steps and ended up experiencing a relapse.

A good example of sequential healing can be illustrated with the example of a fractured ankle. When healing a simple fracture, the vertical line approach is the best way. First the patient is put in a cast, then they do physiotherapy followed by strengthening exercises. After the completion of each step in this sequence, they can go back to a normal life. But if someone with a broken ankle decides to go for a walk after two weeks of being in a cast with the justification that 'walking is healthy', they will compromise this vertical line approach and can risk permanent damage to the injured area.

So follow the simple structure below:

- rest
- repair
- recover
- restore

When you see your healing steps in the above manner, it becomes easier to be patient and the healing becomes foundationally strong. That commitment is something that the warrior has to make to themselves. My protocol works with any autoimmune condition because it doesn't address the symptoms but the root causes. When the root causes disappear, the symptoms fade.

The steps of the vertical ladder of healing are outlined below. I will elaborate on them over the next few chapters.

Step 1: Physical nutrition

This includes what we eat, our physical activity, rest and sleep, how we absorb nutrients and how we release toxins from the body. Nutrition has to be efficiently absorbed inside the body to calm the brain, gut and impacted areas of inflammation. Detoxification via food releases toxins or pathogens and begins to clear the gut, making space to create a flourishing environment for good bacteria to grow and repair the digestive system. For mind-body healing, self-nurturing via the right nutrition is key.

Step 2: Emotional nutrition

This is defined by what we feel, see, hear, absorb, react or respond to. Emotional nutrition balances our emotional sensitivity—or over-reactivity—towards our own thoughts and our environment. We must combine physical nutrition with reduction in reactivity. Yogic calmness breathing techniques achieve a lowered inflammation response while enhancing gut repair, as shown by electroencephalograms (EEGs)—a recording of brain activity—which demonstrated a positive signal when slow breathing experiments were conducted.[1]

Our breath, the *prana*, has to reach a restful state to reduce over-reactivity of the immune system. That is when it can reach a state of stability and gut repair can begin. For when the breath becomes calmer, so does the mind. This cuts the vicious cycle of messages of stress from the brain to the gut and back and gives the gut a chance to begin the healing process. When the mind and body are inflamed, the easiest way to reduce this inflammation is to just pause and breathe.

Step 3: Gut repair

With nutrition and breathing exercises, the mind starts becoming calmer and while the gut repair begins almost immediately, it can take a few weeks to a few months to show results. Signs like clearer skin, higher energy and reduction in constipation indicate that gut healing has begun. The warrior begins to experience more positive moods. These experiences are all linked to gut repair. After this step, the warrior is receptive to moving to the next one, which will bring higher quality of life via movement and mobility.

Step 4: Movement

Why is movement important? The right kind of movement begins releasing tightness and toxins in the fascia—a thin casing of connective tissue—of our muscles and joints. Fascia surrounds and holds every organ, blood vessel, bone, nerve fibre and muscle in place. It has nerves that make it sensitive and provides internal support. When stressed, it tenses.[2] Often the warrior isn't able to figure out whether the pain is in the bone or muscle. This is because of the fascia being stressed and tight due to the autoimmune condition. When our fascia is healthy, it is flexible but when it tightens, it can restrict movement and cause painful health conditions.[3]

This step can be thought of as a 'fascia detox' programme. A combination of yoga and massage therapy, this step is extremely important to start releasing the stress in your fascia. To achieve this, the best form of exercise is slow or restorative yoga. Yoga helps us mediate our stress response, reduces our risk of cardiac disease and improves memory formations.[4] It regulates the parasympathetic nervous system, which is where the vagus nerve is located. When we exercise, do yoga and hold asanas, the fascia starts relaxing, toxins release, the mind and body connect and the signalling of the vagus nerve improves. The warrior will start feeling a release of chronic fatigue when they adapt to slow and restorative yoga. Movement with yoga asanas improves mobility, which is limited when inflammation levels are high.[5]

Step 5: Talk therapy

Also known as counselling, talk therapy is an extremely important step in the healing process. Without us recognizing and releasing subconscious and conscious emotional trauma, we can't move ahead. However, if I try to heal the mind first, the already suffering patient is often not receptive to counselling and conversations as they're too overwhelmed with their poor quality of life. I have seen this frequently in my practice. Only after the warrior attains physical and emotional stability by following the first four steps are they ready to acknowledge and discuss emotional triggers. It's important then to have meaningful conversations about releasing these triggers via therapeutic counselling interventions.

This can be an extremely overwhelming process for them and the counsellor as there are a lot of breakdowns that happen at this stage. It requires a counsellor who is compassionate and understands the autoimmune warrior's mind to be able to help them move ahead. While it is advisable to seek out a certified counsellor, you can also talk to someone you trust who can create a non-judgemental and safe place for you. The purpose of talk therapy is to release your emotions and accept them.

Step 6: New normal

This is the most difficult step because warriors now have to maintain the new homeostasis to cement their healing. At this stage, the warrior starts recognizing that they can dare to hope to get back to normalcy because they're finally experiencing clinical healing. They have never felt this good in a long time. Their self-confidence re-emerges as all their medical tests improve drastically or return to normal ranges.

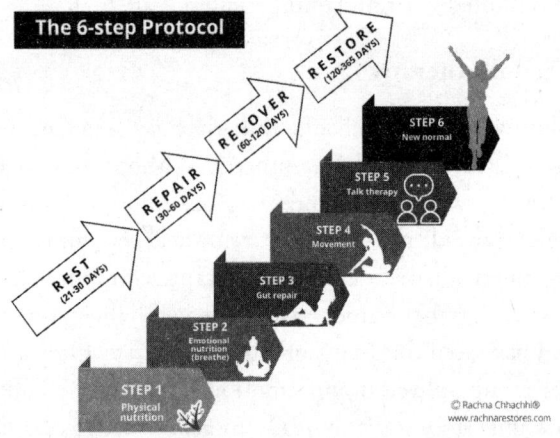

Despite their best efforts, the medical fraternity has failed miserably in understanding the mind of an autoimmune warrior. Whether I look at myself or the warriors I have treated, a large part of my work has been in changing the way our mind perceives the healing. That change can't begin till the foundation of self-nurturing via precise nutrition, breathing, movement and rest doesn't happen. Only after this does the mind get the strength to reject the disease.

In my early days of healing, I was doing all this and getting results. But I was not a certified mental health therapist. I wanted to enhance my own learning to help my patients, so I got certified in mental health therapy. This shifted the clinical impact of my patients' healing and I saw with every patient who healed, that if an autoimmune warrior makes up their mind to heal, there is no stopping them.

6

BEFORE YOU BEGIN

Every autoimmune condition will have specific markers that demonstrate the repair work that needs to be done. Before you start a healing programme, you must get your bloodwork done. Your diagnostics will help you start a clinically evidenced plan and you can monitor your progress through further tests that help you understand how your biomarkers are changing along with your symptoms.

Some of the basic tests that you need to do are:

- **CBC:** To test for low haemoglobin and inflammation.
- **ESR:** A non-specific marker that is usually high during infections. However, in autoimmune warriors, chronic inflammation means that it remains high constantly without presence of active infections.
- **C-reactive protein:** This is also an inflammation marker that is usually used to test for heart disease. In autoimmune conditions, it will be extremely high even without the presence of any other issue.
- **Antibodies**: Please ensure you do the specific one for your condition. However, please add the antinuclear antibody

(ANA) test because a positive ANA is present in many autoimmune conditions. Though it sounds confusing, this test would have been done when your doctor made the diagnosis for your autoimmune condition. So don't worry, just look at your previous reports and you will be able to identify the ones you need to get done. If not, you can get this done yourself. I have seen this positive for most conditions I have treated.

- **Genetic markers:** These include HLA-B27 which is positive in AS, and the other HLAs like B35 for reactive arthritis.[1] You will need to get the one specific to your condition.

- **Liver function profile:** If you have been on medications, your liver is likely to be impacted. This test will show if your liver is sluggish. With or without medications, it is likely to be sluggish.

- **Kidney function profile:** In many autoimmune conditions such as type-1 diabetes and for those who are on medications, keeping an eye on your kidney reports is crucial. Very often the kidneys will not filter out the toxins because the gut and immune system are sluggish. With or without medications, kidney function needs to be monitored.

- **Thyroid profile with antibodies:** Many women with autoimmune conditions can develop a secondary autoimmune condition like Hashimoto's, so it's important to get thyroid antibodies tests done to rule this out.

- **HbA1c:** While this is a diabetes or a haemoglobin sugar marker, we need to keep blood sugar levels low as higher levels increase inflammation in the body.

- **Magnesium:** Low levels of magnesium lead to muscle pain, bone pain, brain fog, nerve pain and fatigue. You will need supplements if your levels are low.

- **Vitamin D:** This is an essential immunity-protecting vitamin and most people have a deficit. However, very high levels are toxic and can lead to kidney damage. This is why vitamin D levels need to be in a healthy range.

- **Vitamin B12:** This vitamin calms and nourishes our nerves. Optimum levels mean reduced pain and better quality of sleep. Healthy B12 levels reduce nerve pain in autoimmune warriors.

7
PHYSICAL NUTRITION

When you begin, even the first step can seem overwhelming. That's because the first step is all about pausing and resting at a time when you have very little strength or motivation to follow a structure. A warrior understands that we can't just jump straight to yoga and exercises because we just don't have the strength yet. Hence, step one of the programme focuses on giving you the strength via a reduction in your symptoms. This step needs to be followed for a period of three to four weeks, depending upon the severity of the symptoms.

But before we take this step, it is important to understand nutrition because there are many misconceptions about it. We often think of nutrition as limited to only what we eat and drink and the supplements we take. But this isn't true. You need to nourish your whole being. Your mind isn't outside your body, and your body parts don't work in isolation. This holistic approach addresses every cell in your body and motivates your mind to follow the path. There are nutrients for the brain that also work for the gut, and approaching nutrition only at the physical level is unscientific. The brain–gut axis is well established in clinical research and medical science. The same foods that calm the brain also calm the gut.

These foods include good fats, probiotics, prebiotics and tryptophan-rich foods such as leafy vegetables, nuts and seeds, oily fish, eggs and dark chocolate. Tryptophan, as we have discussed earlier, is a precursor to the neurotransmitter serotonin, which is a mood-enhancing hormone. Hence, our mental health can also be improved with consumption of the right foods. We will often come across examples of how the mind and body are connected during the healing process. We can't separate them if we want to experience deep inner healing.

THE FIRST STEP—ELIMINATION

The first step is the process of elimination. Some foods that are otherwise considered 'healthy' may need to go. For example, spinach and tomatoes are healthy foods, but they're unsuitable for autoimmune patients because they increase purine levels in the body, thereby increasing pain. This example shows how a generic 'healthy diet' programme can be detrimental for an autoimmune warrior's healing.

The aim is to have 85 per cent of what you eat as plant-based food. As we move through the programme, we can add animal protein only in the form of chicken breast, oily fish and eggs. But we have to ensure it is in small quantities. Now, why do we need to eliminate so many items? It's because the path for healing needs to be clear and uncomplicated. Via elimination, we focus on foods that provide optimal gut health, which is one of the crucial focus areas of the healing process.

Most autoimmune patients have a leaky gut, and with poor emotional immunity and high anxiety, the gut is ravaged. If we continue to eat foods that irritate the gut, then we can't expect a smooth and consistent path to heal ourselves. Remember, you must not even take a bite of these foods. We have to completely and ruthlessly eliminate all the following foods for one full year.

1. Sour items

Many warriors ask me why they need to elimiate sour foods from their diet. Don't they contain vitamin C, which is good for us? Yes, of course they do. But your gut is compromised and hurting, so we need to heal it first. When your skin is bruised, if you put some lemon juice on it, won't it get irritated? Just like our external skin, we also have a skin layer that lines the gut. If you eat sour items, the gut 'skin' which is already corroded due to the leaky gut, will be constantly irritated and can't heal. Also, sour items increase bone pain.[1] Most autoimmune patients have some form of pain, so we need to reduce pain as a part of the treatment. Anything that triggers pain is out.

Here are a few sour items that must be completely eliminated from your diet:

- lime/lemon
- vinegar
- tomatoes
- tamarind
- all citrus fruits
- sour pickles
- fermented foods
- anything sour or tangy

2. Vegetables that interfere with gut absorption

In my practice, I have seen certain vegetables interfere with gut absorption and cause discomfort. Many of these are also on the 'warning list' of the Arthritis Foundation,[2] which publishes scientific literature on inflammatory foods and joint pain.

The vegetables to avoid are:

- eggplant (*baingan*)
- okra/ladies' finger (*bhindi*)
- bitter gourd (*karela*)
- capsicum/bell peppers
- spinach
- corn[3]

3. High purine foods

Purines are naturally found in some foods and produce a waste product called uric acid. A pile-up of uric acid crystals in joints causes gout, joint pain and kidney issues, and can lead to inflammation and pain.

Here are some foods that have been proven by research to increase purine levels:[4]

- lentils
- mushrooms
- seafood
- legumes
- red meat[5]

4. Dairy and fat

We must eliminate all dairy products, including yoghurt. Milk can also increase inflammation because of saturated fat, high mucus levels, lactose sugar and due to the animal hormones in milk interfering with human hormones. A clear link between hormones and fluctuations in pain and fatigue levels can be seen when women experience an increase in inflammation levels a few days before their periods. Dairy products have been shown to interfere with female hormones[6] and hence, all milk products should be avoided.

Once the immune system is healed and stable, you can reintroduce some dairy such as yoghurt and cheese—fermented dairy products—into your diet. When I say 'a little bit', I do really mean a very small amount. If you start having a glass of milk every day, your inflammation levels will start rising again.

Fats to avoid:
- saturated fat such as coconut oil, milk and animal-milk products
- refined vegetables oils (rice bran oil is a lesser devil)
- trans fats, found in packaged foods, bakery products, fried foods and margarine

5. Gluten

When I tell my patients to go off wheat, many of them ask if they're allergic to gluten. They may or may not be allergic, but the issue is more about how gluten reacts in our body. As per a report in *European Medical Journal*, human enzymes can't effectively digest gluten proteins and 'these proteins have been reported to possess differential immune targets that make them immuno-toxic by nature.'[7] The report also discusses at length the negative impact of chemicals and fertilisers that further degrade the quality of wheat. In most places, the wheat that we consume today is primarily made from genetically modified (GMO) seeds, even if the wheat is organic.

For those who don't have an issue with their immunity or have a healthy gut, consumption of wheat in moderate quantities isn't a problem. However, for autoimmune warriors the gut is compromised and healing needs to be done via the gut. Wheat will hinder the healing process.

Hence, the following should be eliminated:

- wheat
- white flour
- oats
- rye
- semolina
- barley

6. Conflict foods

There are some foods that don't work for some warriors while they work for others. These are potatoes, chicken breast, fish, eggs and dark chocolate. If you can find a caffeine-free and dairy-free dark chocolate, you can have it occasionally. After the first phase, eggs and fish are recommended as they contain protein and nutrients that reduce chronic fatigue and brain fog. Most patients I have treated adapt very quickly to eggs as a protein because this type of protein is bioavailable and possesses antibacterial and immunity-protecting properties.[8]

Omega-3 fatty acids present in oily fish has anti-inflammatory properties.[9] In a large study, daily supplements of vitamin D and omega-3 fatty acids resulted in reduced risk and symptoms of autoimmune disease.[10] Oil of omega-3 is also present in walnuts and flaxseeds; however, walnuts are difficult to digest in the initial stages and can irritate the gut, and flaxseed oil isn't as effective. Consumption of omega-3 fish oil has the most protective benefits for warriors. Yes, some patients can't have eggs, chicken and fish because they're vegetarian. However, vegetarian replacements do not have the same impact on chronic fatigue, and fatigue triggers flare-ups. There are times when I go completely vegetarian, but even during those times I make sure that I consume my fish oil supplements. I also increase my quantities of peas, which are a good source of vegetarian protein.

Many warriors can eat potatoes without any side effects but for a few, this can increase gut discomfort or bone pain. Please tune in to your body like I did in the initial stages of my healing. After eating any of these conflict foods, wait for forty-eight hours to see if there is any increased inflammation or other undesirable symptoms. If there are any, eliminate these conflict foods. Otherwise, you can continue to enjoy them. I love my potatoes!

7. Tea, coffee and other sources of caffeine

All of these need to go.[11]

'What is left for us to eat? You have eliminated everything … we will starve!'

This is the usual response I get when I discuss my programme with warriors. However, when I share the actual healing plan, they understand that the conventional norms of what is healthy and unhealthy don't apply to us. Everyone has been brought up with notions of what is 'healthy' and there is now so much information clutter on the internet and social media that even search engines can't always provide clinically evidenced information.

THE PILLS OF LIFE

Along with eliminating specific foods, we need to add supplements. Nutritional supplements are part of the physical and emotional nutrition plan because your gut isn't absorbing enough nutrients from food. This lowers physical immunity and increases adrenal fatigue. Nutritional supplements are necessary not just to support the gut but to also reduce a high stress response. Nutrients such as fish oil help us reduce stress but may not be available in food if you don't eat oily fish. Even vegetarians can take a fish-oil supplement in capsule form. Supplements also help with low serotonin and adrenaline levels.

Here I'll explain the purpose of each of the supplements I prescribe. You need to take the supplements below for at least one year for stabilization and increased absorption. They will strengthen your physical and emotional immunity.

	Supplement name	Purpose	Dosage
1.	Probiotic that has three strains: lactobacillus, acidophilus and saccharomyces boulardii.	Repairs the gut.	One capsule before breakfast.
2.	L-glutathione	Makes the liver work efficiently and reduces fatigue.	500 mg after breakfast.

	Supplement name	**Purpose**	**Dosage**
3.	Ashwagandha	Reduces fatigue and helps with hypothyroidism.	500 mg after lunch.
4.	Milk thistle	Makes the liver work efficiently.	500 mg before dinner. If you have fatty liver, this should be taken before lunch and dinner.
5.	Omega-3 from fish oil	Decreases inflammation, reduces anxiety, repairs and lubricates eyes if they become dry.	1,000 mg after lunch.
6.	Multivitamin with 15 mg zinc	Protects immunity.	One tablet after lunch.
7.	Vitamin E	Protects immunity, eyes and liver health.	400 IU after lunch.
8.	Vitamin D	Protects immunity and bone health and modulates gene expression.[12]	2000 IU after lunch. Increase to 5000 IU if deficit. Don't take injections as extremely high doses put a load on kidneys.

	Supplement name	Purpose	Dosage
9.	Vitamin C	Protects immunity, has antioxidant properties, reduces inflammation, increases production of collagen and reduces anxiety.	500 mg three times a day after meals.
10.	Folic acid	Reduces inflammation and pain.[13]	5 mg after lunch (skip on methotrexate days).
11.	Magnesium	Reduces pain and fatigue, calms the gut, prevents constipation and aids sleep.	200 mg twice a day, once after lunch and once before bed.
12.	Calcium citrate	Strengthens bones and calms the gut.	1,000 mg before bed (taken together with magnesium).
13.	Primrose oil (for women)	Balances hormones.	1,000 mg before bed.
14.	Kelp and L-Tyrosine	Improves thyroid health.	200 mg each after lunch.

	Supplement name	Purpose	Dosage
15.	Glucosamine along with chondroitin and methylsulfonyl-methane (MSM)	Reduces joint pain and swelling, helps with gut repair, increases flexibility, strengthens synovial fluid in joints.	1,000 mg twice a day, after breakfast and lunch.
16.	B vitamins with B12	If you are deficit as per blood report. Don't take injections.	500 mcg B12 with a B vitamin after lunch.

Note: Dosages for children under twelve years are half of the quantities listed above. If the child is below the age of six, it would be a 25 per cent dose.

Many patients ask me if they can get their nutrition only from food and not have all these pills. My answer is no. There are four main reasons for this. They are:

- **The gut of an autoimmune patient is leaky.** Even the most nutritious food isn't going to have optimal absorption since the gut is compromised and needs to be repaired.

- **Autoimmune patients have chronic anxiety.** When your emotional immunity is suppressed, you carry your anxiety with you. For example, warriors with IBS have 'twice the odds of having a generalized anxiety disorder at some point in their lives when compared to peers without the disease,' according to a study.[14] Anxiety reduces absorption of nutrients from food.

- **Autoimmune patients need mood enhancing hormones.** For us to get better, our body needs to start producing the hormones that can reduce fatigue to give us more energy and motivate us. This can be achieved through a combination of food and supplements but can't be fulfilled only with food.

- **Toxins like pollutants, chemicals and stress (stress is an emotional toxin) work like 'anti-nutrients', harming and damaging our body.** Chemicals play havoc with the gut and reduce absorption of nutrients. They are present everywhere—in food, water, the air we breathe and our homes. Our daily stressors don't go away and only become worse with our feelings of inadequacy and emotional vulnerability. Supplements can help to counter the harmful effects of these.

Despite the benefits, many warriors resist taking supplements. I would like to categorically state that in my clinically evidenced healing, it's the combination of nutrition and supplements that works. Don't think of them as pills, rather as the nutrients you're not able to consume or absorb via food alone.

Below are some frequently asked questions about supplements.

Q. Why are there so many supplements?

A. The answers are in the four points listed above. Over and above this, just like some people are prone to gaining weight much more than others, warriors are prone to having a weaker physical and emotional immunity. Supplements keep the supply of nutrients steady in the bloodstream to decrease fatigue and stabilize the nutrition required for healing and reducing inflammation.

Q. Are there any side effects?

A. When the immune system is compromised, we all need additional nutrients. I have been taking supplements since I gave up toxic medications to begin my healing journey. I have observed that if I miss even a week of my supplements, I start feeling fluctuations in my well-being. A higher quality of life isn't achieved by medications but through supplements. So no, for the quantities and how they have to be taken as listed in this book, there are no side effects unless you consume a low-quality brand which has more fillers or artificial ingredients in it. To avoid this, look for organic products, read the labels and purchase your products from high-quality nutrition brands which have higher reviews on various websites.

Q. Do I have to have supplements all my life?

A. Yes. Unless you live on your own farm with no stress and breathe fresh pollution-free air and eat organic food, supplements are for life. The exceptions are vitamin D and B12, dosages of which need to be adjusted every three months as the levels need to remain optimal. This can be evaluated by your doctor or nutritionist.

THE ROLE OF WATER

Water is an extremely important factor in the physical nutrition step. It makes up most of our body. We need water to absorb nutrients and release toxins. Increasing the amount of water we drink can reduce brain fog and also, ironically, reduce water retention because of its diuretic properties. It may sound contradictory, but it is true. Water not only benefits us when we drink it, but also when used for therapy to release pain. Remember: when you feel unwell, 70 per cent of you is water. Less water can induce low moods as brain cells get dehydrated faster.

I have listed here various uses of water for your holistic healing journey and the precautions to take.

Type of water

We live in a toxic world. Very often the water in our pipes at home contains heavy metals, arsenic and other toxins. These toxins can get easily absorbed when we bathe with this water or drink it. Check your water source and use a water purifier not just for drinking but also for bathwater.

Water consumption

The ideal rate at which to drink water is 200 ml every ninety minutes we're awake. Drinking less than this amount can lead to constipation, poor circulation, low metabolic rate and slow absorption of nutrients. Bathing twice a day helps to bring down body temperature and reduce inflammation. It also increases circulation, reduces brain fog and helps us sleep better.

Water therapy

Swimming in winter has been shown to significantly decrease tension and fatigue, boost memory and mood as well as relieve pain.[15] Cold water therapy has been clinically proven to reduce inflammation levels. Research has shown that it reduces complaints of somatic pain in patients with autoimmune disease. This is thought to be a result of a decrease in cellular microinflammation.[16] So if you feel inflamed and in pain, try using cold water instead of having a hot bath. Of course, you need to avoid it if you live in colder climes.

Icing to reduce inflammation

In case you have any injury or inflammation in joints like wrists, ankles, knees or elbows, icing is recognized as more effective than using a hot-water bottle. After resting the joint, apply a cold compress to slow down the excess production of synovial fluid and stimulate sensory receptors to decrease transmissions of pain signals to the brain. An ice or cold pack—a gel one is best—can then be applied for ten to fifteen minutes at a time. You can repeat it up to ten times a day on the inflamed joint. Ice therapy is effective almost immediately and can bring back mobility to the joint if done for three to four days.

8

EMOTIONAL NUTRITION

What we feel, see, hear, absorb, react to, or respond to also affects us and produces a reaction in our body and mind. We have all experienced how emotions impact us physically—we get butterflies in our stomach before a date or an interview or our mouth waters simply by thinking of one of our favourite foods. These are physical behaviours, but they're triggered by a thought process. That is the power of emotion—it can change your response to your external environment.

Soothing emotional nutrition reduces our emotional sensitivity towards ourselves and our external environment. When physical nutrition is combined with a reduction in reactivity to external triggers (which can increase inflammation), the food we eat is absorbed faster by the gut. Even if we're eating well, if there is stress or anxiety, this absorption process is compromised. With calming breathwork, the gut begins absorbing more. Clinically, calming breathwork with music has been shown to repair the gut faster and release anxiety. Repair is also evidenced at the DNA level.[1]

ANULOM VILOM, OR ALTERNATE NOSTRIL BREATHING

Many studies have proven that alternate nostril breathing techniques like anulom vilom or *nadi shodhana* reduce inflammation levels.[2] Although the two techniques are slightly different, their impact on inflammation is similar. For most warriors, anulom vilom works better than nadi shodhana. When the mind and body are inflamed, the easiest way to reduce this inflammation is to just pause and breathe.

I have listed the steps for specific breathing techniques below. You need to do them for the duration listed for the specific phase. You can watch my videos on my YouTube channel, RachnaRestores, for a visual guide. The methodology I follow for pranayama is different from other yoga teachers' because mine is focused on reducing chronic inflammation. I prescribe breathwork for a longer duration and the frequency of breathing exercises is also much higher in my programme.

Remember, doing this pranayama is 50 per cent of your healing process. Prana is our life force and those who can master regulating their breath will have lower pain and inflammation levels, brain fog and fatigue, and will experience a higher quality of life.

With regular practice, alternate nostril breathing has extraordinary health benefits. Within three weeks, you will begin to experience calmness and positivity and your pulse rate and blood pressure will drop. These exercises reduce inflammation and repair your gut. Over a period of time, your prana will begin reducing your symptoms and start repairing the gut. Follow the below steps for maximum impact:

- Do this on an empty stomach. The best time is first thing in the morning or three hours after lunch.
- Sit in a comfortable position with your back straight and knees straight out so that there is no knee discomfort. Support your back, but don't slouch, sit straight. For

those with extreme pain, starting out on the bed is best as the spine is supported, knees are stretched, and pillows can support the arm that helps open and close the nostrils during the alternate nostril breathing.

- Always begin with the left nostril. Use your right thumb to close your right nostril. Then, inhale slowly and deeply to fill your lungs. The inhalation should not be forceful; it should be gentle but deep. Inhalation should be for four seconds. Hold for a second. Now, lift your thumb, close the left nostril with your ring finger and exhale slowly and softly from the right nostril. Exhalation should be for eight seconds and should be gentle, unhurried and flowing. Initially, if you are a beginner, you can focus on exhalation at six seconds, but increase it to eight seconds over a few weeks and maintain that. A good way to do this is to visualize your breath going from your lower back via spine to head, and when you exhale, visualize the breath travelling from your head towards the front of your body, travelling finally to the feet. When you imagine this, automatically the four–eight cycle gets established.

- Inhale again from the right nostril in the same gentle manner, hold for a second and exhale deeply and evenly from the left nostril. If you are a heart patient, don't hold your breath. For everybody else, this is beneficial.

- Inhale again from the left and hold for a second, and exhale from the right.

- Repeat this cycle for five minutes—slowly, deeply, without hurrying. Remember: hurry is your enemy.

- After five minutes, take a couple of sips of water. Repeat the cycle.

- On the first day, only do five minutes. Increase the session by two minutes every day until you get to twenty minutes. From then onwards, do twenty minutes each time.
- Always end on the left nostril. That is our *chandra* or moon, or *ida*, hence 'cooling' nostril and responsible for dousing inflammation. The right nostril symbolizes our *surya* or *pingla*, hence the heating side. Alternate nostril breathing helps us balance both sides and the first and the last inhalation from the left nostril activates our cooling side hence reducing inflammation levels.
- If your arms get tired, use pillows to support them.
- For people with chronic anxiety or depression, this should be repeated twice a day: once in the morning after waking and again at 5 p.m. If you find it difficult to sleep at night or you wake up in the middle of the night, you can again do this breathing to calm and balance your left and right sides so that you release the fluctuations of the mind and, within five minutes, you will start feeling sleepy again.

BHRAMARI, OR HUMMING BEE

Regular practice of humming helps to reduce brain fog and your brain will soon start feeling fresher. This improves your motivation, and you will feel more agile. The humming bee technique also eases brain inflammation—which is common in autoimmune patients—and improves quality of sleep.

- Close your mouth and keep the teeth slightly apart. Position the tip of your tongue to the top palate behind the top front teeth. Make sure to maintain this position of the mouth throughout the practice while ensuring that the jaw remains relaxed.

- Close each ear with the thumbs, place index fingers at midpoint of the forehead—just above the eyebrows—reach the middle, ring, and little fingers across the eyes so that the tips press gently against the bridge of the nose.
- Now, take a long, deep breath in through the nostrils, bringing the breath all the way into the belly. Begin to exhale slowly, making a steady, low-pitched 'ommmmmmmm' sound at the back of the throat—like the humming of a bee. Focus on releasing the breath with the emphasis on mmmmmm. The positioning of the tongue encourages the vibration to resonate throughout your brain, cleansing and rejuvenating it. Focus your awareness to the centre of your head; you need to let the sound fill your brain and feel the vibrations on the sides of your face.
- Begin with five long repetitions. Slowly build this up to ten. As you practice daily, you will realize that each repetition or exhalation of breath becomes longer. Ideally, each repetition should be for about a minute. This can be achieved after a month of daily practice.
- If you feel claustrophobic, don't close your ears and eyes. Just inhale deeply from your stomach and exhale to the sound ommmmmmmmmm. This is equally effective.

Both these breathing exercises need to be done in the order listed above. The ideal mix is twenty minutes of anulom vilom and ten minutes of humming bee, but you need to build up to that level.

DIAPHRAGMATIC BREATHING

Diaphragmatic breathing is called 'belly breathing' or 'abdominal breathing'. Our diaphragm is a large, dome-shaped muscle right below the lungs. The abdominal muscles help move the diaphragm and increase our capacity to empty our lungs. Many warriors experience a dull pain in this area. Diaphragmatic breathing helps you use the diaphragm effectively to reduce this pain.

It also lowers your anxiety levels and heart rate, strengthens the abdominal muscles and aids sleep. If you are one of those warriors who tosses and turns and is unable to fall sleep, this breathing technique will help you doze off. You will also wake up experiencing less pain and better energy levels.

Diaphragmatic breathing technique (lying down):
Follow the steps below just before sleeping:

- Lie in bed on your back, with your knees bent and head supported.
- Use a pillow under your knees to support your legs. This will help you to feel your diaphragm rise up and down as you breathe.
- Breathe in slowly through the nose, you will feel your stomach rise, causing your hand to rise but remain in position.
- Release your stomach muscles, so that your stomach moves in, your hand lowers as you exhale.
- The hand on your upper chest remains as still as possible.

- Continue this for ten deep breaths at the beginning and build it up to thirty or forty breaths. Keep counting your breath as you do the breathing technique until you fall asleep.

Diaphragmatic breathing technique (sitting):

Sometimes anxiety can strike during the day. At such a time, you can do diaphragmatic breathing while sitting in a chair or on a sofa. Follow these steps:

- Sit comfortably with your knees bent and your shoulders, head and neck relaxed.

- Put one hand on your chest and the other on your stomach. This will help you feel your diaphragm rise up and down as you breathe.

- Breathe in slowly through your nose. Feel your stomach rise while your hand rises but remains in position.

- Release your stomach muscles, so that your stomach moves back in, as you exhale to a count of five. The hand on your upper chest must remain as still as possible.

As per Cleveland Clinic, this breathing technique is a wonderful way to reduce anxiety.[3]

I recommend doing breathing exercises daily because stress and anxiety in warriors is always high. These breathing techniques will lower stress, improve digestion, reduce fatigue and improve your sleep.

9
MUSIC FOR PRANAYAMA

Music can be a form of emotional communication that brings together the various parts of your mind and body. Musical activity produces significant changes in the immune system and has a positive impact on various immune-response biomarkers such as leukocytes, cytokines, immunoglobulins and hormones, as well as on neurotransmitters associated with immune response. Music as treatment is now taken seriously in healthcare as research findings have begun to link the beneficial impact of music to a broader influence on our health.[1]

Soothing meditative music helps the brain relax. Combined with deep-breathing exercises, it can result in lowered inflammation levels. When the brain is relaxed, it sends a calming and soothing signal to your gut, thereby aiding gut repair. Hence, music paired with the breathing exercises outlined in the previous chapter is integral to healing the gut. Without music, the results are only half as good.

I have listed below some YouTube channels that have healing music to accompany your breathing exercises. Make sure you keep a glass of water near you and then sit on the sofa or bed. Get comfortable and ensure that your back and knees are supported before you begin. Then switch on the magic of music and combine it with the pranayama to help you heal.

Name of YouTube channel	Name of specific video
Healing Tree Music	'Braincell Activation Music'
Dream Sounds	'Relaxing Music with Ocean Waves at Night'
Healing Soul	'Beautiful Relaxing Music'
Soothing Relaxation	'Flying: Relaxing Sleep Music'
Soundings of the Planet	'One Hour of Perfect Yoga Music'
Mindset	'Cells Healing: Affirmation'
Relax Daily	'Peaceful Mind'
Yellow Brick Cinema	'Relaxing Piano Music'
Soothing Relaxation	'Relaxing Piano Music: Romantic Music'

10

GUT REPAIR

One of the key organs that aids gut repair is the liver. With continuous detoxification of the liver, pathogens can't survive in the gut. The liver's involvement in autoimmune conditions is clinically established.[1] Asymptomatic liver enlargement and elevation of liver function tests is commonly seen even if the autoimmune condition isn't related to the liver. If the condition is connected to the liver, its enzyme readings can be very high.

This happened with Yusuf Aaji, forty-three, from Riyadh, Saudi Arabia. Yusuf was diagnosed with primary sclerosing cholangitis (PSC), a chronic liver disease in which the bile ducts inside and outside the liver get inflamed and scarred and eventually narrow or become blocked.[2] When this happens, bile builds up in the liver and causes further liver damage. The prognosis is usually liver failure, and a liver transplant becomes necessary when doctors can't keep the disease from getting worse.

Yusuf had already been on a nutrition plan for a few months when he came to me. His liver test report results showed that his SGOT was 131 (the normal range is up to 40), SGPT was 489 (normal up to 41), alkaline phosphatase was 338 (normal up to 126), GGT was 1284 (normal up to 61), and bilirubin was 13 (normal up to 7). However, after thirty days of following my protocol, his SGOT and SGPT came down to 29, alkaline phosphatase reduced to 77, GGT to 51 and bilirubin to 9. His autoimmune scores were also high. He had high ASMA 1:100, and high IgG 3 0,97. Both came back to normal with my treatment, the IgG went down to 0.004. He repeated his liver FibroScan to test fibrosis (thickening or scarring of tissues), which had been positive a year ago. And now, it was negative—his liver fibrosis had disappeared!

We did a video session after he received the report. Yusuf was sitting in his car because he didn't have any privacy in his office. And he was laughing. 'I feel fresher, lighter and have more energy,' he told me. 'Earlier I used to get tired by late afternoon, but not now.' He said that it was difficult to adapt to the plan because he had never eaten like that. He had gone to a local nutritionist in Riyadh who put him on a 'liver-friendly' diet, but his reports didn't show improvement and neither did he feel better. 'Frankly, I didn't expect results like this in just thirty days,' said Yusuf. 'I am quite amazed. I am looking forward to getting rid of this disease.' All his reports and scans are now negative for PSC.

One of the early symptoms of an autoimmune condition is chronic fatigue. Doctors and clinical researchers feel mystified by chronic fatigue syndrome, a condition where even regular activities like bathing or walking around the house can lead to debilitating fatigue that doesn't go away with rest. All warriors are familiar with this situation. Yusuf had also experienced this. His energy levels were very low when he signed up.

As per clinicians, there are no known triggers for this fatigue. But Cornell University researchers report that they have identified 'biological markers of the disease in gut bacteria and inflammatory microbial agents in the blood.'[3] This means that your chronic fatigue is in your gut and liver. Bad bacteria in the blood trigger an immune response, which can worsen symptoms for autoimmune warriors.

Rest and sleep douses the flare-up fire

We need proper rest and sleep for the gut to have the energy to repair. Evidence shows that gut microbiota is closely connected to sleep.[4] Abnormal sleep patterns and shorter duration of sleep impact the gut microbiota negatively. Since we need good gut microbiota to repair the gut, rest and sleep become an essential pillar of treatment. The commonly held notion of getting up early in the morning to exercise doesn't work for autoimmune warriors. I have seen early mornings making symptoms worse not just for me but all the warriors I treat. And the moment they sleep it out till late morning, they begin feeling fresher and more agile.

It's only towards the early morning hours that warriors begin to get good sleep. Thus, sleeping in and waking up late in the morning gives them the rest they need to start repairing their gut microbes. This is something unique to my treatment and I have seen it impact the speed of recovery. With all the warriors I've treated, including myself, good quality morning sleep has worked wonders in decreasing fatigue levels. When the warrior doesn't sleep in the morning hours, I notice more flare-ups and poor healing.

Many warriors try to sleep early but are unable to get restful sleep. At this time, I recommend diaphragmatic breathing to ease them into sleep. Sometimes, those unable to practise it wake up early in the morning in desperation and try to exercise. This triggers chronic fatigue through the day and can cause a flare-up if the habit of waking up early and exercising is continued. For regular people, going for a walk is healthy. However, if an autoimmune patient has a flare-up, rest and sleep are the most effective options as this immediately calms the gut microbiota and starts repairing it.

Over the past few decades, it has been proven that the gut is more than just a digestive organ; it also regulates immunity and affects brain function.[5] If the brain has 100 million neurons, the gut contains more than 500 million, making it a powerful partner to the brain to increase immunity, reduce inflammation levels and aid recovery.

Autoimmune warriors have low energy—and this limited resource needs to be channelized into repairing the gut. This makes rest an important pillar of healing.[6] Whether you are starting my protocol or are completely healthy, just remember that if you get a flare-up, rest for forty-eight hours. You will be able to avoid making it worse and eventually the symptoms will recede.

However, if you seek medical intervention during the time of the flare-up, your toxic load will increase from the extra medication, putting more pressure on the gut. This is detrimental to the healing process. In the first stage of healing, rest is paramount. Optimal nutrition in combination with pranayama and music triggers the digestive system to begin restoration. Many warriors who don't rest during this time tend to compromise their healing and their journey takes longer.

SLEEP HYGIENE

'Sleep hygiene' refers to healthy habits and a restful environment that aids a good night's sleep. Improved sleep isn't an overnight process and won't happen as soon as changes are made. But consistently following good sleep hygiene each night allows the brain to break previous patterns of anxiety that disrupt the sleep process. It then adapts to a newer pattern that enhances sleep quality and duration.

Follow the steps below to improve your sleep hygiene:

- Avoid a heavy dinner, coffee or alcohol before bedtime. Eat dinner by 7 p.m. so that the food is digested by the time you go to bed. Caffeine isn't allowed in my protocol but if you still choose to continue having caffeine, don't have it after 5 p.m. Among alcoholic drinks, only red wine is allowed after one month of the programme. If you drink red wine, don't have it close to bedtime, and keep the quantity limited to 150 ml.

- Doing pranayama before bedtime can help you fall asleep more easily at night. In case you wake up in the middle of the night, just focus on diaphragmatic breathing and you will fall asleep again.

- Go to bed every day by 10 p.m. After a few days, your brain will start looking forward to being in bed by that time. You may not fall asleep immediately, but you will start feeling drowsy and restful and eventually doze off by 11 p.m.

- Make sure your bedroom is calm, quiet, dark and relaxing and at a comfortable temperature.

- Restful essential oils can relieve stress. Lavender in particular can improve sleep quality. You can keep a diffuser in your bedroom and allow the fragrance to start relaxing your mind and body.

- After you get into bed, put on some meditative music to help you unwind.
- Chamomile tea relaxes the nerves and calms the gut; drink a cup at bedtime.
- Remove all electronic devices—including phones, TVs and computers—from your bedroom. Not only do they distract, their ultraviolet rays can disrupt sleep patterns.

Do this every day consistently, and within four weeks the brain and body will be tuned to the new routine of peaceful time just before bed. When done daily, these simple habits can transform your sleep pattern, helping you sleep better and longer.

I aim for nine hours of sleep at night. I'm usually in bed by 10 or 11 p.m. and at 8 a.m. the next morning I wake up rested and refreshed. This particular step will impact your healing very quickly and help you recover faster because it works on two levels—it repairs your gut bacteria, and it helps decrease chronic fatigue.

11

MOVEMENT

In the first phase of healing, you can't exercise at all, no matter what. However, you may be surprised to find that you will still lose weight. This happens because breathing exercises calm hormones and release physical and emotional toxins. Often, a lot of our stubborn excess weight is due to fluctuating hormones which can upset the somatic nervous system and hold in toxins. Within thirty days, consistent pranayama combined with the nutrition plan helps to release these toxins and calm the nervous system, making you feel lighter and fresher.

You will experience reduced bloating and, in many cases, also lose a couple of kilos. In some cases, my patients have lost as much as 4 kg, however, if you're already at an ideal weight, don't worry—you'll regain any lost weight back. The mind and body have their ways to reset only up to the level of the balance required. Excess weight is a toxin; if you have that, you will lose it.

After the first phase, it's important to introduce movement to bring in mobility. This movement addresses the following:

- releases fascia toxins
- releases stress in fascia

- increases circulation
- decreases inflammation and pain
- reduces aches and pains
- strengthens joints
- strengthens spine
- increases agility
- increases energy
- improves balance

The movement stage has four phases. The four phases take us step-by-step from being inflamed, rigid or immobile to being flexible and agile with higher energy. It's like preparing for a marathon—we don't just start running. If we do that, we can end up with injuries. Marathoners take up to a year to prepare for the race. It requires discipline and consistency to acclimatize and strengthen the muscles to reach the required levels of endurance and mobility. Respected sportspersons often talk about the role of rest and nutrition in their journey to high performance.

It's important to remember that every warrior is different. For example, some may not be ready to begin yoga as they won't have the strength to hold an asana. For us warriors, it can be extremely difficult initially to include exercises for mobility. We have to take it slow. While you continue with the nutrition and pranayama steps, you can begin the mobility phases listed below. The four phases will gently help you reach the stage where you can experience an agile and energetic life.

PHASE 1

Day 1 to 30: only pranayama

Even though it may be difficult for you to believe, pranayama is reducing your inflammation levels and preparing your mind and body to start physical activity. For the first thirty days, just practise consistent pranayama three to four times a day. It helps you create the foundation for exercise—decreased pain and a relaxed gut. Only then is your body and mind ready to move to the next phase.

PHASE 2

Day 31 to 60: in-bed mobility exercises

In-bed mobility exercises are part of the first step towards achieving increased mobility without straining your joints, muscles and spine. Long periods of standing lead to fatigue in warriors, so lying down for the initial exercises results in less strain and fatigue while still retaining the benefits.

Position: Lie down on a bed or a thick carpet, *not* on a yoga mat. Your joints and body don't have the strength for the mat yet. The bed is best at this stage.

Do the following exercises as described.

Wrist rotation

Many warriors experience pain in their wrists and hands. To decrease this pain and increase circulation, we need to rotate the joint. Even if you don't have wrist pain, remember that your wrist affects your elbow, shoulders and even your spine—so if any of these parts are sore or hurting, wrist rotations are required.

They have to be done slowly and gently for them to be effective. For those with swollen wrists, hold one wrist with the other hand to support it while you do the rotations.

- Sit on your bed or a chair, with your arms extended in front of you.
- Hold your right wrist with your left hand if it's swollen. Gently rotate the right wrist clockwise ten times, and then anti-clockwise another ten times. The movement should be slow.
- Switch sides and repeat.

Ankle rotations

Just like our wrists, our ankles also become stiff due to inflammation, pain or poor circulation. Ankles represent the stability of the foot and by extension the entire body. If your knees are affected, your ankles are likely to be weak.

Doing regular ankle rotations will strengthen the muscles, increase circulation and reduce pain and inflammation in the knees, ankles and feet.

- Sit straight in a chair or at the edge of a bed. Stretch your left leg in front of you, and slowly rotate your left ankle clockwise ten times.
- Then rotate the same ankle anti-clockwise ten times.
- Relax your left leg, then repeat the movement with your right ankle.

Alternative movement:

- In case you are not able to rotate your ankles, you can put your right ankle up on your left knee in a sitting position and use your hands to gently rotate your ankles clockwise and anti-clockwise ten times.
- Do the same with your left ankle.

With the support of the knee and your hands slowly rotating the ankles, they will start opening up and you will be able to do regular ankle rotations in a few days.

Spine twist

The spine is the channel of energy. It has all the nerve signals to the brain and controls body balance. The spine is one of the most important focus areas for autoimmune healing. Very often, warriors have 'root chakra' imbalance because of which the tailbone and lower back hurts.

As we strengthen the spine during the healing process, avoid typing on the phone, laptop or computer or tasks like driving and cooking because all these actions use the shoulders and arms. This can increase pain levels in the upper spine, arms and hands.

Follow the steps below to stretch the spine.

- Lie flat on your back on the bed and draw your knees in to your chest. Don't force the movement—draw them in gently only as much as you can while still being comfortable.
- Slowly drop your bent legs to the left side of your body, feeling a twist in the opposite side.
- Simultaneously, turn your face to the right side (the side opposite to the one your knees are facing). Press your left

hand on top of your knees and extend your right arm to the side at shoulder height for a deeper stretch.
- Breathe deeply three to five times while holding the stretch.
- Switch sides and repeat.
- If your knees don't touch the bed when lowering them to the side, don't force them to. Place a pillow or cushion underneath and lower them only as far as you comfortably can. With time and practice, your knees will touch the bed without effort.

Shoulder and upper arm release

Some warriors experience constant pain in the shoulders and upper arms. The muscles of these areas need to be strengthened by increasing circulation and stretching them out. We can also get pain in the armpits if the lymph nodes in that area are inflamed. For women, the pain areas are usually on the side of the breasts and below them.

When done consistently, this specific exercise will decrease these pains.

- Lie down on your left side and completely extend both your arms in front of your face. The palms of the hands should be touching each other.
- Keep your legs bent at the knees.
- Move your right arm without moving your body, lifting and then taking it towards the opposite side in a semicircle. Try to bring it all the way to touch the bed behind you. This is a slow and gentle movement. Bring the arm back

to touch the palm of the other hand. Repeat twenty times on this side.

- Now lie on your right and do the semi-circular movement twenty times with the left arm.

After this exercise, you will immediately feel your shoulders, arms and upper back opening up. For many, the first few repetitions will be difficult and cause pain. But keep going, because as the circulation increases, the pain will decrease.

Butterfly pose

The butterfly pose—or *badhkonasana* and its variant, lying down *bhadrasana*—stretches the hips. Most warriors have stiff hips, which is a common cause of poor mobility and agility. Hence this is a very important pose to open your hips and bring back your agility.

- Lying face-up on the bed, turn the soles of your feet in to touch each other. Allow your knees to fall away from each other, opening up your groin area.
- If your knees don't touch the bed, you can put cushions or pillows under each knee and rest your knees on them.
- Focus on breathing deeply for three to five minutes while holding this pose.
- Practice this pose daily for seven to ten days. After ten days, progress to the following steps.
- Lie for five minutes in the butterfly pose with your soles touching, and then bring your knees together to touch each other.

- Lower again to the original butterfly position.
- Gently repeat this up-and-down movement—which represents a butterfly flapping its wings. You can use cushions to support your knees if they don't touch the bed.
- Doing butterfly flaps after holding the pose increases agility and opens up the hips.

Wind pose

The wind pose—or *pawanmuktaasana*—helps the gut heal. It releases excess bloating or wind in a gentle manner, giving relief to the abdominal area.

- Lie on your back and draw your knees up towards your chest. Don't put additional pressure on the knees if they're hurting—bend only as far as is comfortable.
- Wrap your arms around your legs below your knees and touch your forehead to your knees if possible. If not, hold your shins as comfortably as you can.
- Take five long, slow, deep breaths.
- On the last exhale, release your shins and lower your knees.
- Repeat five times.

Do all the exercises in Phase 2 both in the morning and evening and you will start feeling your agility and freshness increase. You may hear cracking sounds from your joints when you're doing these exercises—this is normal.

Soon you will be able to get out of bed or up from the floor much more easily. Continue with these exercises indefinitely

PHASE 3

Day 61 to 90: mobility exercises

Calf strengthening

- Sit on a chair. Now raise your toes to tighten your calves. Hold for ten seconds and then release. Repeat ten times in the morning and evening.
- After doing the sitting calf-strengthening exercise for seven days, try to do it standing up. You may be able to stay on your feet only for one second, and that is fine.

Remember to do the standing exercise on a soft padded surface only and not directly on the floor. This will further increase your agility and balance.

Lying-down cycling

This strengthens your knees, gut muscles and legs.

- Lie down on your back and extend your right leg completely while folding your left leg against your abdomen. Keep your hands on your sides or under you, supporting your lower back.
- Release the left leg while you fold and bring the right leg closer to your abdomen. The left leg should now be straight and the toes pointing outward.
- Repeat this cycling motion ten times initially and build it up over a period of three weeks to thirty repetitions.

Side stretches

Side stretches are important to open your hips and strengthen your legs. For most warriors, poor balance and feeling wobbly are common. Strengthening the legs will ensure that they don't buckle under.

- Lie down on your left side. Fold your left leg at the knee.
- Lift your right leg till your toes are pointing towards the ceiling.
- Bring it down to your side. Repeat ten times.
- Switch to the opposite side.
- Over a period of two weeks, build it up to thirty repetitions on each side.

Stick pose

The stick pose—or *yashtikasana*—releases fatigue. End your daily exercises with this pose. It reduces the inflammation of the lymph nodes, increases circulation and boosts immunity.

- Lie down completely straight on your back with your arms by your side.
- Inhaling deeply, stretch your arms above your head while keeping them in line with your body.
- Stretch the body to its full length. The toes and the fingers should be stretching in opposite directions.
- Maintain the stretched position for a few seconds while holding your breath.
- Exhale slowly and return to the starting position. Relax the hands and toes.

- Repeat three times.

- After three rounds, keep lying in the starting position with your eyes closed for five minutes. You can then get up and do your pranayama.

The benefits of natural surroundings

You may not yet be ready for a full-fledged walk even if you feel you are. Instead, try walking barefoot on grass for ten minutes. This gives you the additional benefits of 'earthing', also known as 'grounding'. Research shows that direct contact with the earth's surface transfers energy from the ground into the body and produces anti-inflammatory effects.[1]

Also, exposure to healthy microbes (including bacteria and fungi) found in natural areas can reduce inflammation and give us immunoregulatory benefits.[2] Let's utilize these benefits to reduce inflammation levels by stepping out into nature whenever we can. This could even be in a community park near us.

Breathing exercises done in natural surroundings stimulates healing. Carry your headphones with you and listen to soothing music while you do your breathing exercises. Being close to nature automatically brings down inflammation levels.

PHASE 4

Day 90 onwards: add restorative yoga

The differences between regular yoga and restorative yoga can be found in the intensity and pace. Restorative yoga emphasizes gentle, supported postures held for extended periods, which in turn starts to release the fascia tension and toxins. Depending on the style, regular yoga often involves more dynamic movements, active poses and transitions, which are challenging for those with pain and chronic fatigue. Restorative yoga, on the other hand, uses props for support, like blankets, cushions and blocks to support the body in each asana, providing a sense of comfort and ease. Even though props are used in a regular yoga class too, the emphasis there is on building strength and flexibility, which is too demanding for those with autoimmune disease at this stage.

Restorative yoga aims at triggering the relaxation response, promoting calmness and reducing stress. A regular yoga class also includes relaxation elements, but the emphasis is mainly on physical exertion. Energy conservation is one of the factors that makes a restorative yoga class more suitable for those with pain and chronic fatigue as it's designed to conserve energy and promote rest.

Prachi Wasnikar, forty-three, has been a restorative yoga and immersion teacher since 2016. She lives in Amsterdam and works with warriors struggling with pain and sleep issues. 'The gentle and supportive nature of restorative yoga makes it appealing for those looking for a practice that can help manage pain and promote relaxation,' she explains. 'I often have students with autoimmune conditions experiencing pain. Restorative yoga offers a space for them to engage in gentle movements and relaxation techniques, helping them manage symptoms better.' Prachi's experience of working with autoimmune patients has shown her that consistent practice can have positive effects on pain relief and sleep quality.

While individual responses vary, most of her participants have experienced reduction in stiffness through the gentle and supported postures that help release tension in the muscles and joints. Many also see an improved mind–body connection, as mindfulness and breath awareness in restorative yoga contributes to a heightened sense of body awareness. This increased awareness helps individuals manage and alleviate pain by recognizing and addressing areas of tension. Another frequent result is better sleep, as the calming and restful nature of restorative yoga contributes to improved sleep quality over time.

Prachi recommends adding the three asanas below to your healing programme for maximum benefits. You can start with these and then look for a restorative yoga class near you, which may also help you connect with other warriors.

Supported Child's Pose (Balasana)

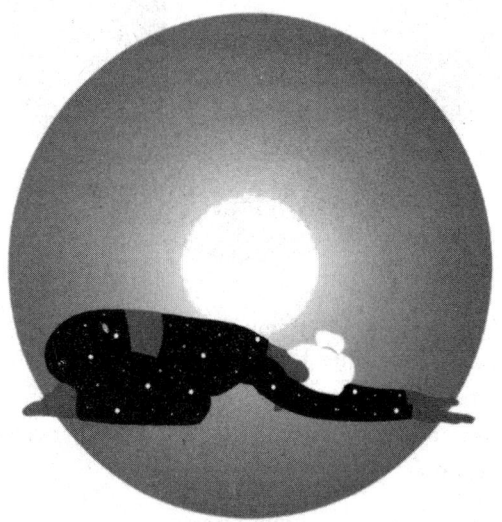

How to do it: Start in a kneeling position, then lower the upper body forward, extending the arms in front or alongside the body. Place a bolster or stacked blankets under the torso for support. Focus on your breath flowing in and out of your body and rest in the pose for anywhere between five and twenty minutes.

Benefits: This pose gently opens the lower spine, hips and thighs, promoting relaxation and releasing stress in the spine.

Legs up the Wall (Viparita Karani)

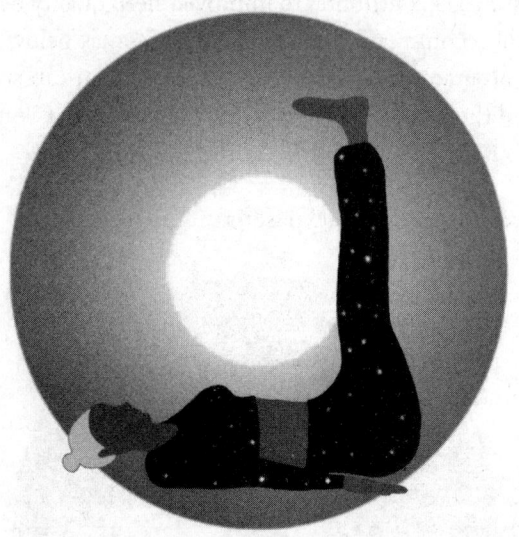

How to do it: Sit close to a wall, then lie on your back and gently place your legs up against the wall. Place a folded blanket under the hips for support. Focus on your breath flowing in and out of your body and rest in the pose for anywhere between five and twenty minutes.

Benefits: This inversion helps improve circulation, reduces swelling in the legs and encourages a sense of relaxation, alleviating fatigue.

Supported Reclining Twist

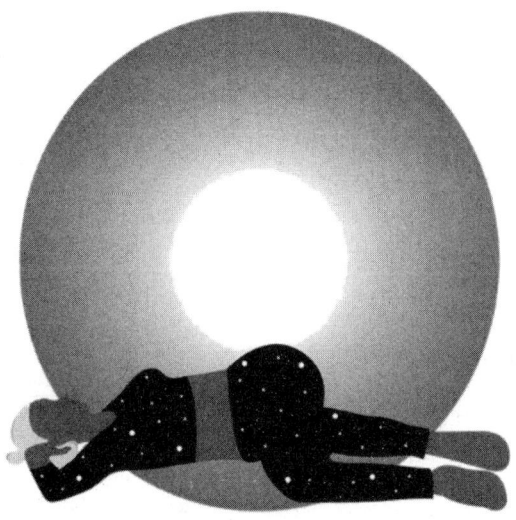

How to do it: Lie on your back with knees bent. Shift the hips slightly to one side and drop the knees to the opposite side. Put a thin bolster or a folded towel under the knees for support. Repeat on the other side.

Make this a thirty-minute sequence for a well-rounded set as it addresses different areas of the body and enhances an overall restorative experience. Listen to your body, use props for support as needed and consult with healthcare providers if you have specific health considerations.

Benefits: This movement gently stretches the spine, shoulders and hips, promoting relaxation and releasing tension in the back.

Summary

All this can feel confusing since you're adding exercises at different stages. To help you, here is a convenient table with a summary of the exercises you need to do at each stage.

Day 0–30	Day 31–60	Day 61–90	New Normal
Only pranayama	Ankle rotations	Ankle rotations	Ankle rotations
	Wrist rotations	Wrist rotations	Wrist rotations
	Spine twist	Spine twist	Spine twist
	Shoulder and upper arm release	Shoulder and upper arm release	Shoulder and upper arm release
	Butterfly pose	Butterfly pose	Butterfly pose
	Wind pose	Wind pose	Wind pose
	Pranayama	Calf-strengthening exercises	Calf-strengthening exercises
		Lying-down cycling	Lying-down cycling
		Side stretches	Side stretches
		Stick pose	Stick pose
		Walk on the grass	Balasana
		Do your pranayama in nature	Legs up the wall

Day 0–30	Day 31–60	Day 61–90	New Normal
			Supported reclining twist
			Walk on the grass
			Do your pranayama in nature

By the time you begin restorative yoga, you should be feeling almost normal. But remember, for one year you shouldn't overdo exercise. Everything has to remain nurturing and in balance. Go slow and preserve your energy so that even during exercise you don't cause oxidative stress and invite a relapse. The combination of exercises given above, combined with the restorative yoga asanas and breathing exercises, will create your foundation of healing.

For the first year, we need to combine all these elements consistently without any interruptions to derail us. Those who don't take this seriously often have a relapse from trying too much too soon. For one year you need to be patient with yourself and kind to your body and mind to nurture your immune system in its recovery process. This wonderful body is your vehicle for fulfilling your dreams. Keep it nurtured, stable and agile. It will support you in your daily activities, your travel, your fun times and in rest.

Never forget to rest when you feel tired. There will be days when you feel completely exhausted. On those days, only do pranayama. Skip the exercises. Try to do the exercises at least five days a week so that your circulation and agility can keep improving and your joints and muscles can keep getting stronger.

COMMON QUESTIONS ABOUT EXERCISE

Q. Why can't I go for a walk when I start the healing programme? Walking is healthy.

A. When we repair the gut to get the strength to absorb nutrients, the digestive system takes up a lot of energy. If we allot that energy towards physical exercise, the process of beginning the repair work is compromised. Also walking until the spine, hips, leg muscles and joints are not strong can cause fatigue and flare-ups. The exercises in Phases 2 and 3 will help strengthen the lower part of your body to prepare you for normal walking.

Q. After I am fine, why can't I go to the gym?

A. Any form of exercise which is heavy leads to oxidative stress. Oxidative stress increases inflammation levels even in normal people, but recovery from oxidative stress is faster if it's combined with periods of rest. For an autoimmune patient, oxidative stress increases inflammation levels and antibodies. Going to the gym also means you will be supervised by someone who may not understand what limitations you have and can lead to injury of the already damaged joints or spine. Moderate exercise such as the given stretches, restorative yoga and moderately paced walks (after six months) is recommended.

Q. I need to build my muscles and strengthen my joints with weights. I have been told that weight training is best for this.

A. Absolutely right. But keep in mind that yoga is a weight-bearing exercise—you use your own body's weight. That is why yoga asanas can build that muscle and strengthen your joints. Lifting dead weights can trigger fatigue. This is something I have experienced myself and with warriors I have treated. But doing bodyweight-bearing exercises under the supervision of a qualified yoga teacher ensures that your joints and muscles are being strengthened in synchronization with your mind. After finishing a few months of my protocol, you can join a regular yoga class. That is a better way to achieve your desired aim.

Q. How do I keep my fascia free of stress and toxins?

A. The focus of all the phases of mobility that I have given is the release of toxins and stress from the fascia. When we have a cleansed fascia, we experience a higher level of agility. Continuing with the movement protocol in this book as a lifestyle modification for the rest of your life will ensure that your fascia is strong, cleansed and stress-free, helping you be pain-free, supple and mentally fresh.

12

TALK THERAPY

Talk therapy, or counselling, is the fifth step in my healing protocol. At this stage, it's as important to seek out a good counsellor as it is for you to become your own counsellor. The first three weeks are spent in pacifying the agitated mind and gut. The elimination diet, supplements and pranayama blend with each other to reduce brain agitation, repair the gut and bring about the first signs of healing in the form of freshness and lowered pain levels. When we introduce movement, suddenly we start discovering that our clumsy and imbalanced body can be sprightly and dexterous. There is a liveliness that starts arising in our demeanour.

At stage 1, the warrior is angry. They feel powerless and are unable to make decisions because their brain is foggy, their body is weak and their spirit is broken. The anger begins to fade by the time we reach the 'movement' step in the vertical ladder of healing. And that's when a conversation with oneself or others is helpful in moving forward. Once the magic of nutrition and pranayama has begun to show results, the warrior is ready to have a calmer conversation about their emotional triggers. They have realized that they do have a chance at a normal life. At this stage, talk therapy will help the warrior reach the next level of healing to release their emotional toxins.

Many warriors don't address emotional triggers and hence it takes them longer to heal. I understand this since it took me a long time to accept that I had emotional triggers. I never thought I would need counselling. That is our mindset, and breaking this mindset is an important step towards healing ourselves. The caregiver or healer must provide a safe counselling space and continue the healing beyond the superficial level. If we acknowledge our triggers and fears and accept our limitations as well as our positive traits, we can be at peace with ourselves. Crying and talking about what you have never talked about helps to address the triggers. The counsellor can support you through this process.

I did talk therapy with my mother much later in life. Long after I had healed my RA, I still held anger about my childhood experiences. But after many rounds of heart-to-heart conversations with my mother, our bond became even stronger. I understood her struggles as a wife, which I needed to do to let go of the loneliness of my childhood. We had eight good years of talking and laughing until she passed away.

At this stage, conversations with oneself or someone you consider a safe space can create a bigger impact in emotional healing. Suddenly you can see how far you have come and start believing in your own self-worth. This is the time to express your feelings by journalling and doing some introspection to reach a stage of clarity and emotional balance. The graph below will help you reflect and understand that you always have a choice. Exercise that choice.

COUNSELLING FOR SELF

THINGS OUT OF MY CONTROL	VS	THINGS IN MY CONTROL
The past		How to nurture myself
Other people's attitudes		Deep breathing to let go
The future		Manifesting a positive future
What others think of me		How I think of me
Other people's opinion based on their life		Creating my self worth
Toxic people		Defining my boundaries

Forgiveness for self—and/or others—can't be embraced till all these are addressed.

It's not always easy to create a safe space to ease one's emotional triggers. I remember one of my RA patients in Chennai was so angry with her father, but she couldn't have a conversation with him because he was no more. So, I suggested that she close her eyes and have the conversations she wanted to have with him as if he were present in front of her. This helped her let the past go. But this self-healing isn't possible for everyone. Sometimes, we need a professional counsellor to hold our hand and emotionally nurture us in releasing our emotional toxins.

I have listed some self-care techniques in this book, but you must find someone you can have a conversation with. You could talk to a trusted loved one who you feel is neutral territory. Below are some of the things to keep in mind before you start therapy.

Accept that you need talk therapy

It's important to have a non-judgemental person to talk to. This is a crucial step in your healing journey. Embrace and accept the fact that talking to someone is going to help you. Sometimes we don't even know we need a counsellor. Kamal Brar of Seattle made that mistake and suffered a relapse of her ulcerative colitis as a result of stress from her emotional triggers.

Understand the difference between a counsellor and a therapist

Both counsellors and therapists help with emotional support. A counsellor offers clinical support for mental health illnesses or a specific type of trauma. If you feel you have a history of mental illness or trauma, you must reach out to a counsellor. A therapist has a more holistic approach and can support you for a longer period, which is what most warriors need since we have conditions that are chronic.

Often, the counsellor will provide the support you need but the therapist will have strong communication skills and an understanding of your emotional health, and can offer a lot of useful tips, resources and structures on how you can help ease your emotional triggers. In other words, a therapist offers a *therapeutic* approach to healing.

It's okay not to know what to say in the first session

We may not be ready to talk about our triggers with a therapist, or we may just release our emotions in the very first session. My experience with autoimmune warriors is that many of them cry in the first session. This starts helping them release their pent-up emotions and that is a huge step in the healing process. The reason most of my patients are able to share their innermost emotions and fears is because they know that I have been through a similar experience myself. That makes them feel that they're on safe and non-judgemental ground. If this resonates with you, look for a therapist in your area with personal experience of autoimmune disease. It may be easier for you to start sharing your feelings at the outset. You can also seek out a support group for talk therapy.

Be regular and consistent

It's easy to feel healed pretty quickly, especially when you are following the holistic nutrition, pranayama and exercises. Our endorphins and serotonin levels start rising, making us feel good. However, the emotional work will not be complete for a long time. Look for a counsellor, therapist or other safe person who can be connected to you for at least six months.

If you have several emotional triggers, seek out a professional counsellor. Don't quit counselling for at least six months. This will provide stability to the physical and emotional immune system. Emotional triggers can cause a relapse. Addressed systematically over a six-month period or longer, they become manageable and our reactivity to them starts reducing.

PART 3

A nourishing meal soothes the soul as it regenerates and restores the mind and body.

13

PHASE 1—DAY ZERO TO THIRTY

THE DETOX

There are many warriors who don't get better even after trying many kinds of nutritional programmes from top doctors and therapists. It's because you can't get results from only generic anti-inflammatory foods for physical nutrition and fermented foods for gut healing.

Nikhita Dadmi, a college student from Bengaluru, found this out when she was diagnosed with psoriasis and was told that there's no cure for her disease.

'One day I looked into the mirror and noticed some dandruff-like stuff on my head,' she recalls. 'Having self-diagnosed it as dandruff, I looked for home remedies to cure it. I found mild relief but a week later the dandruff came back. A bit worried, I consulted a doctor.' That's when she was diagnosed. The doctor told her that she could only manage the symptoms. Nikhita tried many kinds of nutritional plans but imagine a teenage girl being told that there was no cure for this. 'I was terrified. I came home and researched psoriasis and realized that the condition I was suffering from was "autoimmune", where the immune system is triggered and mistakenly attacks healthy cells. To cure myself from this debilitating condition, I approached allopathic and homeopathic doctors. Nothing seemed to work. I was 50 per cent covered in scales, fatigued, sleepless, depressed and went into a loop of self-pity. I had reached rock bottom.'

For Nikhita, psoriasis also came with low self-worth issues because it's visible to others. A young girl is often led by her confidence and Nikhita had lost that because of everything she had read about this condition online. But after only ten days of following my programme, she began to see results. Within two months, most of her skin lesions had disappeared.

Before you embark on your new nutrition plan, remember that you mustn't skip meals. With fatigue already present, doing things like intermittent fasting or not eating till noon is going to make you feel even more tired. It will also throw your hormones off and increase fatigue and pain. Breakfast is very important, especially for those with a thyroid issue. It's the balance of nourishment throughout the day that will give you strength.

The importance of rest can't be overemphasized during the first month of a new nutritional plan. Switch off from work, people, exercise—anything that interferes with the healing process. When you follow the plan, you follow it almost in isolation. Ideally, don't do any other activity apart from what is in my programme. Your energy is being utilized to repair your gut instead of being wasted in activities that will dissipate this energy. The digestive system takes a lot of energy to start healing itself. If we don't rest at this stage, gut healing will not get triggered. So follow the programme exactly as listed. The only other activities you need to do are for personal hygiene, such as going to the washroom. You should also have a bath, preferably twice a day.

It's important to carefully follow the recipes in this book because they're part of clean eating, and always remember to use whole spices, not powders. They are very concentrated in powder form and can cause discomfort in the gut. There are no packet masalas used in meal plans; even home-ground spices are not allowed because these can cause discomfort and put a load on the gut as they're in the concentrated form in the powder. Except for organic turmeric and black pepper, which can be ground at home, whole spices for tempering, such as cumin, mustard, fenugreek, cloves and cardamom are good to have. You can also use curry leaves and herbs such as oregano, thyme and rosemary. Feel free to flavour your food with whole, clean ingredients in their *natural* form.

ABOUT EVOO

Extra-virgin olive oil is a must. I've had many discussions about this with patients who would rather use desi ghee. EVOO may not be native to India, but it is shown to have anti-inflammatory, gut-calming properties. That is why EVOO is the main ingredient in the healing Mediterranean diet that is gaining popularity across the world. Research confirms that EVOO is beneficial for immunocompromised patients, as it contributes to the reduction of the typical symptoms of autoimmune disorders.

The protective effects of dietary EVOO supplementation can be seen in a reduction of inflammation in gut mucosa in chronic colitis.[1] EVOO's anti-inflammatory and anti-arthritic properties are proven to be beneficial for RA, psoriatic arthritis, AS and other arthritic autoimmune conditions. The oil has demonstrated immunomodulatory properties in primary and secondary prevention and management of SLE, osteoarthritis (OA), MS and other forms of sclerosis.

A diet enriched with EVOO improved pathological findings and deferred the disease onset in ALS and neuro-degenerative diseases by increasing motor performance of muscle-fibre areas.[2] The research has proven that the consumption of EVOO and its minor constituents is very important in nutritional therapy, especially in immunocompromised patients. It provides an alternative approach for the prevention and management of different inflammatory diseases.

How to spot quality olive oil

Trust your senses. Real olive oil should smell and taste bright, peppery, earthy or grassy. It could even be a combination of these. Fresh, original olive oils will have a bright flavour with a peppery bite. The pepperiness is from the presence of polyphenols. Fake olive oil might taste greasy, rancid, flavourless or plain unpleasant. A green colour usually means a robust-tasting oil that gives your throat a pleasant tickle when you swallow it. Many patients mistake this for throat irritation if they're not used to the taste. If the EVOO is irritating your throat, it's authentic.

Most genuine producers sell EVOO in glass bottles. Plastic or metal containers can leach toxins from the surface and adulterate the olive oil. It's important that the oil is protected from light and air, which can cause it to deteriorate and spoil. There is also a spurious olive oil industry, but they usually don't use glass bottles as these bottles are more expensive and easier to break than plastic ones.

Look for producers that have third-party testing done on their oils and report the findings, including data such as the 'polyphenol count and free fatty acid levels, which are important measures of quality. Look for a seal from a third-party certifier, such as the California Olive Oil Council (COOC) or the International Olive Council (IOC).'[3]

The endnotes have references to research on the benefits of EVOO, which also reduces liver issues like fatty liver, helps overweight people lose weight, maintains good gut health and lubricates the gut for regular bowel movements.[4] Good quality olive oil is an essential investment and your *amrit*. I carry my own bottle of olive oil everywhere I go—even to the best restaurants—because I want to be sure of the quality! If you don't like the flavour of olive oil in your food, you can mix two tablespoons of EVOO in two tablespoons of food just before eating and enjoy the rest of the food separately.

How to eat effectively

- **Serve yourself:** Even if you don't cook your own food, you must serve yourself. While serving, whisper a small prayer of gratitude for this food to bless you.

- **Rest immediately after lunch:** It's important to rest immediately after. Lunch is the heaviest meal of the day and if there is complete rest after eating, the absorption of nutrients is higher, which increases the rate of repair in the gut. For better digestion, lie on your left side because the left side of our body contains yin energy, which nurtures us. When we lie on this side, the digestive system gets nurtured. If you can't lie down, sit in a reclining posture and listen to some soft music. Meditation music will help you digest food better and increase good microbiomes.[5]

- **Don't skip any step:** Sometimes it can get tempting to skip a few steps but even if you follow only 80 per cent it's not good enough. Remember you have an incurable disease as per medical science, so be true to yourself and follow everything to the dot. Don't short-change yourself because ultimately this is all about nurturing yourself back to good health. And that can't happen if your own commitment is half-hearted.

> **Phase 1 Goals**
>
> - *Detox from inflammation*
> - *Calm the gut*
> - *Reduce fatigue*
> - *Strengthen the liver*
>
> Follow this plan consistently for thirty days. Yes, I know it's boring. In the upcoming steps, your options for food expand and you'll get more recipes. You need to have a repetitive diet only during Phase 1.

THE PLAN—PHASE 1

After waking in the morning, go to the washroom and freshen up. Then consume the following:

- One teaspoon organic turmeric.
- A pinch of black pepper mixed in one teaspoon of EVOO.
- A wholesome probiotic (see p. 64) swallowed with 100–200 ml water that has one tablespoon fresh aloe vera juice dissolved in it (see p. 191 on how to make aloe vera juice at home).

Morning pranayama schedule

Before you sit down to self-nurture with pranayama, play some healing music. This makes the brain calmer and more receptive towards reducing its mental frenzy, allowing you to focus on the breath. Then begin your morning pranayama schedule (see p. 73). Start with a few counts of normal deep breathing by inhaling to a count of four and then exhaling to a count of eight. Repeat ten times, or as many times as you need to feel calm. This is to centre yourself to get prepared for going deep into calming breathwork.

Now begin twenty minutes of anulom vilom followed by five minutes of bhramri.

After pranayama: breakfast

- One wholesome probiotic supplement (see p. 64).
- **Four days a week, alternating:** One bowl poha/rice porridge (sweet or savoury as per your taste). When breakfast is on your plate, put two tablespoons EVOO on it and mix. Do not cook with olive oil.
- **Three days a week, alternating:** One bowl quinoa upma/turmeric risotto—choose as per your taste. When upma/risotto is on your plate, put two tablespoons EVOO on it and mix. Do not cook with olive oil.

One hour later

Have 250 ml of lukewarm water followed by one cup of green tea. Then add a chamomile teabag to the same cup with fresh hot water.

Snack (1 hour later)

At room temperature: smoothie or bowl of six to seven pieces papaya, one apple, ten almonds, ten pistachios.

Half hour later

Have 250 ml of lukewarm water followed by one cup of green tea. Then add a chamomile teabag to the same cup with fresh hot water.

Before lunch

- Ten counts of normal deep breathing—breathe in to a count of four seconds, breathe out to a count of eight seconds. Repeat ten times.
- Practice five minutes of humming bee/bhramri (long exhalations).

Lunch (1-2 hours after snack)

- **Four days a week, alternating:** Overcooked khichadi/stew of white rice or quinoa (quinoa for diabetics or those with high HbA1c, avoid white rice) with vegetables, proportion of veggies to rice after cooking should be 50:50.
- **Three days a week, alternating:** Rotate the three soups below and combine with five to six tablespoons of boiled white rice or quinoa. A word of caution: soup can cause bloating in some. So don't overdo the soup or forget to add the carbohydrates. White rice is a prebiotic so it can calm the gut. Quinoa is easy to digest and rich in protein. Have a small quantity of soup if it causes bloating and combine it with the relevant carbohydrate—white rice or quinoa as per your blood reports. Here are a few soup options:
  - celery and broccoli soup
  - spring onion soup

- mixed vegetables soup

When lunch is on your plate, add two tablespoons of EVOO. Do not cook with it.

After lunch

Rest for an hour while listening to soft music of your choice. Keep your phone away. The left side is our nurturing yin energy. We have to nurture our gut back to good health and afternoon rest is important. If you are working, you can just recline back on your office chair and close your eyes, and listen to meditative music for twenty minutes. Shutting down immediately after lunch is needed for the gut to heal.

Teatime

- A cup of green tea followed by one chamomile teabag/leaves in the same cup with hot water.
- Have this with half pomegranate (seeds) or five to six red/black grapes (whichever is available) and one tablespoon chia seeds (raw).
- Follow this with the supplements listed (see p. 64).

If you feel a little hungry/munchy after having the fruits, you can have the snacks listed below:

- ten pistachios with five tablespoons puffed rice snack (*murmura*).
- ten pistachios with five tablespoon roasted flattened rice snack (*chivda*).
- ten pistachios with ten to fifteen roasted fox nuts (*makhana*).

Before dinner

- One glass of room temperature water, followed by one green and chamomile tea mix as mentioned previously.
- Follow this with music and breathing.
- Now begin twenty minutes of anulom vilom followed by five minutes of bhramri.

Half hour before dinner

One glass of room temperature/lukewarm water.

Dinner (by 7 p.m.)

- **5 minutes before:** One milk thistle.
- **Three days a week, alternating:** Khichadi/stew, similar to what you had for lunch. Use different vegetables though. Add two tablespoons EVOO in the food.
- **Four days a week, alternating:** One bowl of gourd/squash curry or soup, equal quantity of boiled white rice/quinoa. When food is on your plate, add two tablespoons EVOO in the rice. If you don't get gourds, you can use one of the soup recipes from lunch and combine it with your carbohydrates.

9.30 p.m.

Supplements as listed (see p. 64).

10 p.m.

Switch off the lights, lie flat on your back with one hand on you navel, and turn on some meditative music. Focus on the music and your breathwork as listed below and you will dose off soundly.

- Ten counts of diaphragmatic breathing.
- Five minutes of humming bee/bhramri.
- Twenty long counts of diaphragmatic breathing (long exhalations done lying down).
- Sleep.

COMMON ISSUES IN PHASE 1

In this phase, commonly reported issues include bloating, headaches and constipation. Why do these side effects happen? Remember, we're trying to heal the gut, which is trying to adjust to the high nutrients you are giving it. That takes up a lot of energy. Bloating can be reduced with further rest, consistent pranayama and more water intake.

Some of the other 'problems' warriors face during this phase are listed below:

- *You don't consider tomatoes to be 'sour'.* Since tomatoes are generally considered to be healthy, it takes a while to give them up. So, you continue to eat them until you repeatedly remind yourself that they're not part of your programme. Hence it takes longer for Phase 1 to show results.

- *You assume you need to eat bland and boiled food.* This isn't true. In this programme, packet masalas and even home-ground masalas are not allowed because your gut is too weak to absorb the concentrated spices in powdered form. But you can still have whole spices and herbs. Choose these as per your taste.

- *You don't like the taste of olive oil.* You end up reducing the quantity of EVOO as consuming two tablespoons per meal seems 'too much'. However, the combination of olive oil with vegetables is very anti-inflammatory and ensures gut repair. So don't reduce the quantity and definitely don't skip it. As mentioned, you can mix the oil with part of your food at the start of your meal and then enjoy the rest of the dish without it.

- *You miss tea/coffee.* I understand, but you must avoid it because even 'just a bit, without milk' will throw your gut out of order. Be firm in your resolve. Whether black or with milk, tea will mess up your gut and reduce iron absorption. Coffee has been clinically proven to increase inflammation and pain for autoimmune warriors. Both tea and coffee also reduce absorption of nutrients, so you must avoid them completely.

- *You consider breathwork to be an 'additional' or 'optional' step.* Most warriors focus on food for healing. But nutrition is only 50 per cent of your programme. Breathwork is just as important to your healing. The technique, duration and order of breathing exercises must be followed as listed to reduce anxiety and repair the gut.

- *You feel that there is no variety in the food.* This could not be further from the truth! There are only a few vegetables that are not allowed (see p. 60), so you still have a wide choice of vegetables to add variety.

- *You miss wheat.* This is a common complaint when giving up addictive foods, such as the many forms of gluten and dairy.[6] Take heart; there are so many carbohydrates that are going to be included in Phase 2 of this programme that you will feel pampered! Rice—whether white, brown, red or black—as well as quinoa and amaranth will be allowed in any form! But not right now. Don't add them during this phase otherwise your leaky gut will not heal.

- *You find everything repetitive and boring.* Focus on two things:

1. You have taken the first step to heal from an incurable condition. Of course it's going to be difficult, but you're on the path to getting better.
2. If you want different results, you must do things differently. Nurture yourself, be kind and patient with yourself and your body will thank you for it.

14
PHASE 2—DAY THIRTY-ONE TO NINETY

In Phase 1, you have already experienced a shift in healing. This gets stabilized and then is accelerated in Phase 2. The second phase also becomes easier as there is more variety in food choices. Although there are more recipes, the ingredients remain the same. Exercise is also added at this stage, helping warriors strengthen their muscles, loosen their joints and improve circulation.

Phase 2 Goals

- *Stabilize the gut*
- *Release emotional toxins*
- *Improve balance*

Farah Hai is a physiotherapist from London who was diagnosed with RA.

'When the rheumatologist told me that my condition isn't curable, I had no option but to believe her,' she recalls. 'As a physiotherapist, my training and experience with RA patients had also taught me that there was no cure. I had never seen anyone recover from RA. I tried several medications, steroid injections, physiotherapy, acupuncture, homeopathy and herbal medicine, but nothing worked.' Many years of pain and illness led to low self-esteem. Gradually, over time, her RA worsened and she became depressed.

'I had tried so many treatments that holistic healing was just another treatment to try,' Farah admits. 'When you are desperate, you try anything. I will honestly say that I didn't believe that I would ever be free from RA. But holistic treatment saved my life.' Farah believes the change in diet worked first followed by the breathing exercises and yoga. When she finished her detox, her pain levels were nowhere as high as they were when she began the treatment. She says that the diet plan gave her results within a couple of months. 'Be patient, eat according to the phases and you will see results,' she advises.

THE PLAN—PHASE 2

Farah is one of the many who has benefitted from the plan. As you finish your thirty-day detox, remember that the best is yet to come. With that perspective, you can dive into the next few weeks, which will be easier.

After waking in the morning, go to the washroom and freshen up. Then have the following:

- One teaspoon organic turmeric.
- A pinch of black pepper mixed in one teaspoon of EVOO.
- A wholesome probiotic (see p. 64) taken with 100–200 ml water that has one tablespoon fresh aloe vera juice dissolved in it.

Exercise

Do the in-bed mobility exercises as explained in Chapter 11 (Movement). In Phase 2, we only add simple stretches lying on the bed. Your emotional immunity is still fragile, and this is demonstrated by physical rigidity. Follow the phase-wise exercise plan as given in this book. You may feel energetic enough to start going for walks, but don't do it. We are still conserving energy, and any oxidative stress due to exercise can cause a relapse.

Music

Play healing music before you sit down to self-nurture with pranayama. Then begin your morning pranayama schedule. Start with normal deep breathing and repeat ten times, or as many times as you need to feel prepared for going deep into calming breathwork. Now begin twenty minutes of anulom vilom followed by ten minutes of bhramri. Once your pranayama is done, it is time for breakfast.

Breakfast

Eat a wholesome probiotic. Choose options from the section on breakfast recipes. Add two tablespoons EVOO into your food just before eating.

One hour later

Have 250 ml of lukewarm water followed by one cup of green tea. Then add a chamomile teabag to the same cup with fresh hot water.

One hour later

Make a protein powder with almonds, pistachios and chia seeds ground in equal quantities and store it in a glass jar in the refrigerator. Add one tablespoon to a bowl with half a pomegranate (seeds) and six to seven pieces of papaya at room temperature.

Half hour later

Repeat the water–green tea–chamomile tea routine after half an hour.

Before lunch

Do ten counts of normal deep breathing followed by ten minutes of bhramri.

Lunch

Eat lunch one or two hours after your snack. You can choose any one of the options below.

- One to two almond-flour parathas or pancakes with a vegetable curry or stew. Add a salad of cut romaine lettuce with cucumber, onions and one tablespoon of protein powder. Sprinkle salt and pepper to taste and drizzle with two tablespoons of EVOO.

- You can replace the almond-flour parathas or pancakes with vegetable quinoa pulao. Have with the curry or stew and a bowl of romaine lettuce salad with cucumber, onions and two tablespoons of EVOO.

- Add two eggs as you like. Two eggs, with yolk daily, are good for health. Add a few spoons of boiled white rice or quinoa. Have a romaine lettuce salad with cucumber, onions, salt, pepper and two tablespoons of EVOO.
- One to two quinoa rotis, pancakes or a wrap with a large bowl of stir-fried vegetables. You can add half a mashed avocado to your romaine lettuce salad. Don't forget to add the EVOO.

After lunch

Rest for thirty minutes. Listen to some soft music of your choice while resting. Keep your phone in a different room.

5 p.m.

- One apple and ten pistachios with a cup of green tea and then a hot cup of chamomile tea.
- Follow this with the supplements listed (see p. 64).
- If you haven't eaten eggs either for breakfast or for lunch, you will feel fatigued at this time. However, don't eat eggs for dinner as it can cause bloating. Instead have a cup of warm almond milk with one heaped teaspoon of cocoa powder and one heaped teaspoon of protein powder.

6 p.m.

Do the calf-strengthening exercises as explained in the 'Movement' chapter and have a glass of lukewarm water after you finish.

Evening breathing

Begin the pranayama, with ten counts of normal deep breathing followed by twenty minutes of anulom vilom and ten minutes of bhramri.

Dinner

Eat dinner by 7.30 p.m., choosing from one of the options below:

- A bowl of soup from one of the included recipes, combined with boiled brown rice, quinoa or white rice depending on what you feel like (and your blood sugar levels). Don't have soup every day as it can cause bloating. Also don't have the same soup everyday.
- 200 gm oily fish with a portion of vegetables, and a salad that primarily has romaine lettuce, salt, pepper and two tablespoons of EVOO. Add boiled rice or mashed potatoes if you are hungry.
- Replace the fish with chicken breast if you like, keeping the vegetables, salad and rice/potatoes the same as the previous option.
- Any of the rotis or pancakes given in the recipes section with stir-fried vegetables or vegetable curry. Add a couple of tofu or vegetable cutlets—but avoid tofu if you have thyroid issues.
- Chicken or vegetable pulao with vegetable curry.
- Rice noodles or pasta with pesto sauce and stir-fried vegetables.

- Any of the claypot meal options provided in the recipes.
- Simple boiled white rice with vegetable curry.

Important notes:

- The ratio of main dish to vegetables or salad should be 50:50.
- Two tablespoons of EVOO need to be added to all the options just before eating.

9.30 p.m.

In case of constipation (passing stools only once a day is considered constipation), take Softovac powder, which is available online across the world. Dissolve two heaped tablespoons—*not* the green spoons in the bottle—in 250 ml of water. The gap between dinner and this step should be two hours so you should take it at 9.30 p.m if you had eaten dinner by 7.30 p.m. You can take this later if you ate dinner later than prescribed above (which isn't ideal).

This is followed by the supplements before bedtime.

10 p.m.

Switch off the lights. Play some meditative music while lying flat on your back with one hand on your navel. Focus on the music and do your breathwork as below.

- Ten counts of diaphragmatic breathing.
- Five minutes of bhramri.
- Twenty long counts of diaphragmatic breathing.

These steps will help you doze off in a matter of minutes.

THINGS TO KEEP IN MIND DURING PHASE 2

Keep the 85:15 rule

Vegetables, soup, a small quantity of permitted grains and salad must be 85 per cent of your plate. The remaining 15 per cent has to be one of the permitted proteins. This ratio will ensure that all your organs, bones and nerves perform in an optimal manner.

To lose weight

Reduce quantities of grains and carbohydrates and increase quantities of salad. Have the romaine lettuce salad for both lunch and dinner. Don't use any other type of lettuce. If romaine isn't available, you can increase the quantity of stir-fried vegetables (see p. 230).

Eat to nourish

You need to eat till you're 80 per cent full; you should never feel 100 per cent full. Calorie reduction by 20 per cent is linked to the activation of SIRT1 gene, which is our anti-ageing gene and protein. This practice has been evidenced to drastically reduce inflammation levels, ageing process and the risk for lifestyle and degenerative diseases.[1]

Never skip any step

You're nourished in four ways—with food and supplements; with exercise; with breathing exercises; and with rest and sleep. You need all these forms of nourishment simultaneously to heal. None of them are optional or of a lower priority. So please don't skip or modify any of these steps.

Increase protein

Almond milk, almond-flour parathas, green peas, tofu, nuts, eggs, fish and chicken breast are all good sources of protein. Choose from these and consume consistently because your muscles need protein to reduce fatigue. To understand what suits your body, have a protein and wait for forty-eight hours to see if it has aggravated any symptoms. Some warriors don't react well to fish, some to tofu, others to chicken. But the vast majority do not have any adverse reactions at all to these protein options. However, do keep in mind that if you have thyroid issues, you should avoid tofu and soy in any form.

Be mindful of your limited energy

In Phase 2 you will begin to feel more energetic, and you may want to do more—rediscover your life and go out or get into the kitchen and make some amazing food. Don't. You still have limited energy and can relapse and feel fatigued if you don't continue to rest at this time. The only activities you have to focus on are the ones listed previously. Be mindful of this. After a few months, you will be able to do more, and after that you only need to listen to your body. Whenever you feel tired, just rest it out for a day or two and you will be fine.

The physical restrictions are temporary

This isn't how the rest of your life is going to be. You will be able to enjoy yourself and lead a healthy, active and agile life. But just like we need to put a broken ankle in a cast for the required amount of time for it to heal completely, you have to put yourself in a metaphorical cast (this programme) to heal your autoimmune condition.

However, some food changes are permanent

You're beginning to feel better because you have eliminated some of the things and habits that made you unwell. Keep it that way. Anything harmful that you have stopped eating when added back, will make you go back to your previous symptoms and life. Leave your previous life behind and walk ahead. Some things that should never come back into your life are sour items, including tomatoes. After one year of creating a good foundation, some cheat days are allowed. By that time you would have accepted and embraced the food, breathing and movement changes that have been allowing you to heal.

Be grateful for these changes so that they can have a deeper impact on your healing. Every time you feel a craving for foods you want but can't have, remind yourself of the suffering you have been through. That momentary weakness of the tastebuds will pass.

15
PHASE 3—AFTER NINETY DAYS

After three months of following the programme consistently, you suddenly feel almost normal. But you are not yet healed. However, you might want to go out because you have more energy. This phase helps you do exactly that. It gives you the freedom to step out for a meal or plan a trip with loved ones even as you continue the healing process.

Phase 3 Goals

- *Continue the stability*
- *Cement the healing*
- *Increase exercise*
- *Implement your new normal*

Vimi Gupta is an MS warrior from Bengaluru who had childhood trauma from her father's illness. She thinks her eventual trigger was financial and emotional stress. 'After my son was born in 1994, I fell into postpartum depression,' she tells me. 'No one understood it, not even me. After three years, a financial crunch hit our family. That was when the triggers began.' Vimi's case is a classic example of physical and emotional immunity being imbalanced. She was already carrying childhood trauma and then she experienced further triggers.

Vimi says that she isn't as affected by the behaviour of people around her after undergoing holistic treatment for her condition. The breathwork and yoga we do together has reduced her over-reactivity to her environment. She slowly let go of her feelings of anger and frustration and became more stable emotionally. The physical nutrition has helped her get stronger and release toxins from her body.

An autoimmune condition like MS usually comes with the general prognosis of life in a wheelchair. What helped Vimi heal was how engaged she was with the programme. In the initial phases I had to push her, but when she started seeing the results, that was no longer necessary. Even years after her treatment ended, she continued with her new normal of yoga and breathwork. She now eats only pure organic food because her husband started an organic farm after seeing her suffer. The clean eating, yoga and pranayama enhanced her physical and emotional immunity.

You will also experience this shift. At this stage, you will feel cleansed, more physically and mentally agile and some parts of the puzzle of your autoimmune condition will start coming together. You will experience a change and look forward to the bigger variety of foods that you can eat. Eating out becomes easier in this phase.

I encourage you to go out to restaurants after ninety days of following the programme. In fact, eat out once a week. Emotionally, it's good for you because you will make the effort to look nice and dress well when you go out. Women might wear makeup and do their hair. Looking good helps us feel good.

AT THE RESTAURANT

Keep these points in mind when you are eating out:

- *Remember the permitted ingredients:* When you are eating out, always keep permitted ingredients in mind when you order. Specify to the server or chef that you are allergic to sour items so they must not put any lemon, vinegar or tomatoes in your dish. MSG and ginger are also to be excluded.

- *In a Chinese restaurant:* You can order steamed fish or stir-fried tofu and vegetables. Eat it with five to seven tablespoons of steamed rice.

- *In an Italian restaurant:* Order a side portion of salad of only romaine lettuce leaves with grilled fish. Ask them not to add lemon butter sauce. An alternative is Caesar salad with eggs. Ask them to not add the dressing.

- *Always carry EVOO with you* to pour over your vegetables or food at every meal. Even the most luxurious restaurants serve second-press olive oil as EVOO is expensive at this scale. This is true around the world. Therefore, I recommend buying a 100 ml glass bottle of EVOO and always keep it in your bag.

- *Drinking red wine:* Once a week, you can have one or two glasses of red wine. Wine has antibacterial, antiviral and antiparasitic properties,[1] but don't have too much. Enjoy eating out with your loved ones and say cheers!

WHETHER AT HOME OR TRAVELLING, DEVOTEDLY FOLLOW THE TENETS OF PHASE 3

Eat three meals and two snacks daily

This is important to keep your energy constant. If you need to lose weight, you can reduce the quantities—but don't skip any meal or snack.

Always use EVOO

Keep at it, two tablespoons at every meal.

There are more permitted fruits, nuts and seeds

Apple, papaya, pomegranate, red or black grapes, muskmelon, pears and some sweet berries are all okay, but don't have any sour or citrus fruits. If you have thyroid issues, avoid pears. For one year, the only permitted nuts are almonds and pistachios. Walnuts are amazing but they can be a little harsh on the gut. Regarding seeds, only chia seeds and whole spice seeds for tempering were allowed earlier. However, now you can add seeds more liberally, so go ahead and flavour your food with sesame seeds, sunflower seeds or pumpkin seeds!

Continue pranayama and the exercises

Just like your autoimmune condition isn't unidimensional and has multiple symptoms, the healing is also multidimensional.

Nutrition, breath and movement are all pillars of your healing

One without the other doesn't work. So even if you are feeling good, don't skip or add more exercises or foods. At this stage it is even more important to follow this rule because your exercise has increased drastically from when you began. Continuing with this physical activity will help repair and restore your joints and body.

No red meat nor any milk products

For many who relish these foods, this may seem very difficult to follow. Remember, your plate has to be 85 per cent plant-based as the anti-inflammatory power of vegetables is unparalleled with any other food. But you do need animal protein in small quantities to reduce muscle fatigue, so I have provided some recipes using chicken breast and fish. Feel free to come up with your own unique recipes as long as you are not using non-permitted ingredients. Make sure you combine it with a large quantity of vegetables and salad as well as EVOO as this will reduce any negative effects of animal protein and only keep the positive impact.

Continue the supplements

The supplements will keep you on the path of optimal nutrition and will work wonders for your health in combination with the correct food and regular pranayama.

Make time for yourself

Be mindful of this. Your energy has increased and you're physically feeling better, so now you need to start feeling emotionally and mentally engaged. It's a good time to rethink your career choices. If you are not working, you can start exploring something meaningful to do that can make you feel like you have a purpose in life. Waking up every morning with a purpose is important for healing.

Don't overwork

While I strongly encourage every warrior to find purpose in their work, overworking can trigger a flare-up. So those who are in the corporate sector, like I was, may benefit from a transition away from such a hectic life to doing something that gives them joy. Of course, it should also enable them to earn a living. Both are important and linked to self-worth.

Phase 3 is the time for introspection. There are some self-counselling tips provided in the counselling chapter—you can use those to help you find your next calling.

16

YOUR NEW NORMAL

After three months, the first two phases are completed. You will feel much better by now, but of course that depends on how strictly you followed the plan. The perspective with which you approach and embrace the plan is key. However, even if you are feeling better, this is still wet cement. We have to create a strong foundation and it takes one year for the cement of your immune system to dry and become solid.

Rutuja More is an RA warrior from California. When she first sought treatment for her condition, every doctor she consulted would tell her that her reports were within the acceptable range. But her joint pains were getting worse every day. It was only after she searched for a solution on the internet that she found my LinkedIn page and wrote me a desperate message asking for help. After my treatment, her symptoms were resolved.

'I am so grateful for your guidance and I can't thank you enough for guiding me through this and making life fun again,' she wrote to me after she completed my programme. I met Rutuja many years later and found her filled with gratitude for her new life. I try to follow up with most of my patients long after their treatment. I usually find that they have embraced their 'new normal', leaving behind the old lifestyle, stress responses and eating patterns that had led to their disease. This keeps them healed.

You too are now shifting to a new normal.

At this stage, it's very common to deviate and break the guidelines of the programme. Sometimes warriors skip the breathing exercises or overextend themselves at work, or go on a long vacation leaving behind the diet plan or supplements. Don't do things like that. It could lead to a relapse. Give yourself one year to get healed.

YOUR NEW NORMAL

Don't eat what's not allowed

There are very few items on this list. The world is full of other tasty things. Choose to eat what your mind and body deserve and not what will destroy your sense of well-being. Loved ones will nudge you and say you are fine now so you can try something else. Don't. They are not the ones who've suffered. Choose meals and restaurants that allow you to stick to your nutrition plan. Most of the ingredients you're allowed to eat are available around the world. Most restaurants would have a stock of things you can eat. If you discuss your dietary restrictions with them in advance, many restaurants are kind enough to customize a dish for you.

Eat mostly salads and vegetables

Eighty-five per cent of your lunch and dinner should comprise the permitted vegetables and romaine lettuce.

Always add EVOO

As I have highlighted before, EVOO has been proven to preserve joint health, heal the gut, protect the organs, reduce inflammation levels and increase brain freshness. You need all of that consistently. Adding EVOO to your diet will result in good joint lubrication, lower your cholesterol and promote heart, kidneys and liver health.

Add fruits, nuts and green and chamomile tea

Twice a day—between breakfast and lunch and between lunch and dinner—have a snack comprising fruit, nuts, seeds and a cup of tea that has both chamomile and green tea leaves. You can add organic honey if your sugar levels are fine.

Never skip exercises or pranayama

Embrace your exercises and pranayama as lifelong friends and our true healers. We need them to stay healed. Do them wherever you go so that in every situation, you feel great.

Find a purpose

This is very important. When we're restoring ourselves, the first three months are focused inward. But after three months, you start gaining a certain kind of energy along with calmness. You want to put that energy to good use, so find something that makes you feel worthy and useful. Don't work nine-to-five (which ends up being nine-to-eight very often)—that kind of job can invite a relapse. Find something that you can do for a few hours a day so that you wake up with a purpose. However, don't extend yourself so much that you trigger fatigue. After one year of limited work hours, you can increase it to a full day's work, but never tire yourself.

Define your boundaries

Whether you are working, a student or a homemaker, you need to draw boundaries for self-nurturing. This will help you stick to your diet and your schedule for exercise and breathwork even when family members or friends try to push you to skip just one day.

Carry your supplements when travelling

You can get convenient little boxes to store your supplements, which makes it easier to carry them with you everywhere you go.

Remember, we always have a choice. You can choose to continue this new normal and stay healthy or you can choose to mourn all the things that you used to do in your life before the advent of your disease. I stopped cribbing about my previous life when I began appreciating the agility and freshness that I experience today. I no longer look back. Instead, I chose to move ahead and began to focus on what healed me. Make that choice for yourself.

17

MY NORMAL

Many warriors ask me if I still follow everything exactly according to my programme even a decade and a half after healing myself. My answer is yes. To give you a sense of what my 'new normal' is like, I am listing not just what I eat on a daily basis but also the habits, practices and philosophies that keep me healed.

WHAT I EAT

I eat 85 per cent plant-based food. Having said that, I don't miss my 15 per cent animal protein. My primary carbohydrate is potato, and sometimes white rice (but not as often as potato). I eat animal protein in the form of organic eggs or chicken breast and occasionally, fish. I have noted that I could skip animal protein without fatigue until a couple of years ago, but when I hit menopause, my need for animal protein to keep myself nourished is now consistent. Except for breakfast, every meal has vegetables and romaine lettuce. I don't use plates and instead eat out of a medium-sized bowl. This helps me control portions and eat 20 per cent less than my capacity.

I drink three to four cups of green tea daily till about 5 p.m. I use teabags made from cloth or loose leaves to avoid the toxins in regular teabags. I enjoy chamomile tea to feel warm and cosy on cool evenings when I am curled up watching a movie. My day of eating and drinking is in greater detail below.

Breakfast: Nearly always poha and potatoes or potatoes and eggs. If I am travelling outside India I don't find poha, I switch to potatoes. My EVOO bottle is never too far from me, whether I'm at a local restaurant, in another city or even in another country.

Mid-morning snack: Usually lightly roasted salted almonds with a cup of green tea. On other days I may have some papaya or apple instead of the nuts.

Lunch: Always romaine lettuce combined with whatever vegetables are available, with rice or potatoes on the side. Of course, always with two tablespoons of EVOO added.

Late-afternoon snack: A cup of green tea with roasted rice flakes. Sometimes I skip this and eat an early dinner instead.

Dinner: More romaine lettuce with vegetables, but twice a week I add oily fish or chicken breast, very specifically. Rice or potatoes on the side with EVOO added.

Cheats: Cheese, twice a week, with red wine. A couple of bites of bread in a month, because I love eggs Kejriwal and potato-sesame toast. I treat myself to just two bites of these bread-based dishes, once in thirty days.

WHAT KEEPS ME HEALED

More supplements. What I have prescribed in this book is less than what I take, and also less than what I prescribe to autoimmune warriors who come to me for treatment. Because I don't know your entire case history, including specific blood-test reports, what I have prescribed here are the safe quantities to consume even without reports and specific symptoms. I also take higher quantities of vitamin C. I aim for at least 3 gm a day, sometimes taking 5 gm on days I feel tired. I have been following this since the time I healed myself.

Copious amounts of water. I have been accused by my family of drinking too much water. I drink close to four litres a day. I don't count or measure the water; I just drink it every hour or two—even in the middle of the night. It works for me. It keeps my kidneys and liver strong, improves my circulation and efficiently releases toxins. It also keeps my skin healthy.

Stretching. Every couple of hours I get up and stretch. I walk around the house or my clinic or wherever I am. This could be for five or ten minutes. I do this at least four times a day outside of my regular exercise schedule. This improves my circulation and reduces any stiffness I would have otherwise experienced. It keeps me more agile as I grow older.

Yoga and pranayama. I never miss my sessions. Never. Because I have practised yoga, pranayama and dhyana for many years, my resting heart rate ranges between 50 and 55. In comparison, the normal range in healthy people is between 65 and 70, with a lower number indicating better health. I always do evening yoga at 6 p.m. To ensure I don't miss this time, I don't schedule any patient sessions in the evenings. The last session at my clinic starts at 5 p.m. and finishes by 6 p.m. I do yoga after that. It helps me keep my structure of rejuvenating myself with yoga and pranayama before dinner. When I'm travelling, I finish yoga in the morning. This keeps me calm and mentally active. Off late, I have added mild weights to my yoga schedule so that my joints and muscles can remain stable and strong as I age. I have an inner urge that drives me to be agile till the last day of my life. Hence, my weights schedule is focused on building muscles around my damaged joints in my knees, ankles, wrists and shoulders, so that my muscles can support these joints and I can hope to avoid surgical interventions.

Other healers. Doing yoga in isolation at home for years may lead to us getting accustomed to the routine and becoming unable to see if our form is still okay. Periodically, I join a group yoga class to receive feedback from teachers on my flexibility and form. Getting feedback from another yoga teacher helps me understand where I need to improve. I also have conversations with doctors about their observations on triggering healing in patients with similar case histories but different outcomes. These interactions keep me curious, alert and hungry for more knowledge. They inspire me to keep working harder to help others as well as myself.

Studying. I am continuously getting newer certifications to gain more knowledge to help myself and others. At the beginning of every year, I select a course to which I want to dedicate myself to that year. Sometimes it takes longer than a year to finish. But feeding and nourishing my curious mind feels as important as nourishing my body. I am an overthinker, so channelizing my overthinking into a meaningful output has enriched the foundation of my healing.

Being outside. Because of the nature of deskwork, it's extremely easy for many of us to just be in our offices or consumed in studies all day. This has a negative impact on our mental health.[1] I used to feel low in the early days after starting my healing practice. However, once I began stepping out to meet people, or just taking time to work at an outdoor café by the sea, my moods improved. I am at my healthiest and most energetic when I travel.

So don't stay cooped in, especially when you are feeling low or unwell. Just stepping out of your home or office will bring some cheer. Meeting people often reduces social frailty,[2] which is defined as not having too many people or friends to interact with because of your health. This is common in autoimmune warriors and can reduce your self-confidence and upset mental equilibrium. I too had experienced this when I had physically isolated myself and refrained from meeting people, attending events or travelling as I was still healing. However, when I resumed these activities, my social frailty disappeared, and my self-confidence returned.

Escapism. I avoid confrontations. I would rather walk away from an unpleasant situation than try and win an argument while making it ugly for myself and others. When I strongly believe in something, I sit down and explain my point of view and invite the other person to put across theirs so that we can arrive at a consensus. However, if at any point I start feeling like I am not getting through to the person or they start becoming antagonistic, I withdraw. I have done this with family, friends and colleagues.

I am a selective introvert. My peaceful circle only has those people who come from a place of love or compassion and engage in dialogue with reason so that we can talk a matter through calmly instead of being stubborn. I submit to a different perspective if it makes more sense to me. But if we can't understand each other, I disengage instead of getting upset. Because when our peace of mind is disrupted, inflammation and pain strike us. That isn't worth enduring just to win an argument.

PART 4

Attraversiamo, let's cross over.

18

FEELING NORMAL

Rohit Patwari was in his twenties when he was diagnosed with the autoimmune disease called focal segmental glomerulosclerosis (FSGS). It's a rare condition in which the immune system produces 'a chemical that causes the filters in the kidneys to leak. The tiny filters, called glomeruli, become scarred. Scarring often leads to nephrotic syndrome, a disorder where the kidneys excrete extra protein in the urine.' This in turn can lead to progressive renal failure. It's most common in children and teenagers.[1]

Even if treated, FSGS can lead to kidney failure in six to eight years after proteinuria begins. If there's kidney failure, patients need dialysis or a kidney transplant to survive. After suffering for ten years with this condition, Rohit came to me in January 2017. 'Initially I thought it was some infection that would resolve itself in a few days,' he told me. 'But as days went by, my condition worsened.' The doctors first thought that he had membranoproliferative glomerulonephritis (MPGN). He was admitted to a military hospital in immense pain and stayed there for four months with no improvement.

'My body became double my original weight due to water retention, but I could barely eat anything,' recalled Rohit. 'I was on water restriction and was allowed only one glass of water a day. That was when I started feeling that I might not survive this disease.' After three years he had a biopsy and that was when he realized that he had been given a wrong diagnosis. With the correct medication, at first his condition improved. But a couple of years later the side effects of the medicine kicked in and posed a serious threat to his heart.

'A month went by without taking immunosuppressants and all my initial symptoms reappeared,' he told me. 'The doctor advised a kidney transplant and asked my family to prepare for it. That was devastating. In despair, my father reached out to a homeopath. In three months, my symptoms improved with homeopathy.' It was like a miracle and his nephrologist was stunned. He continued homeopathic treatment for two years and began leading a normal life again. However, his condition soon worsened again.

'I knew something was terribly wrong,' said Rohit. 'I felt helpless. There are numerous times when I felt like ending my life because of the extreme suffering. Due to water retention, there was a time when I couldn't drink water even in the peak of summer.' That was when he approached me. However, at the time I had never treated FSGS. I began treatment by going to the root cause of repairing his immune system and gut, with special emphasis on kidney-friendly foods and supplements. Unfortunately, Rohit had already been through so much disappointment that he was sceptical about my programme.

'The programme had things I had never heard of or never thought I would have to quit,' he admitted. 'So many supplements, eggs daily, no legume, no wheat, no tomatoes, no raw nuts! I quit within a week, telling myself that this wouldn't work.' He had stopped emailing me by April 2017.

But he was back in December of the same year, by which time his weakness had reached its peak and he could barely get out of bed. He had stopped going to his office and was working from home permanently. 'I knew I couldn't live like this,' said Rohit. 'I restarted the programme with a determined mind.' Once he started to see improvements, he kept going.

His improvements in a matter of a few months are listed below:

Before my treatment, Rohit's symptoms included:	After my treatment, Rohit felt improvements in the following ways:
Acute chronic fatigue to the point of being unable to perform daily chores. He couldn't drive or leave home.	Reduction in fatigue. Could do daily chores, work, travel and drive.
Brain fog.	Brain fog disappeared.
Extreme spikes in pain in knee joints.	Knee pain totally gone.
Extreme itchiness in legs and shoulders.	Itchiness totally gone.
Blackish texture on scalp.	Scalp normal.

His reports soon began to show clinical evidence of improvement. By early 2018, I could encourage Rohit to step out of his home again. He had been homebound for such a long time that it was impacting his self-confidence. The only way to help him move ahead emotionally was to get him to do things he thought he could never again. He first went on a trip to Jammu, his hometown. When that went well, he became confident enough to travel to the United States the next year.

Rohit got his life back. He now lives and works in Georgia in the US. He is a happy, energetic father and has a flourishing career. 'One thing I've realized after following the protocol for the past five years is that without discipline, we can't make much progress in improving our health,' pointed out Rohit, saying that once you see the programme working, you will automatically get the required self-motivation to continue following it.

When we self-nurture, the body heals. That's what happened with Rohit. His prognosis was poor, but he didn't accept it as his fate. When you are following this protocol consistently for a few months, you will begin to feel the same. You will get your life back too. Embrace the change. It doesn't start immediately.

EMBRACE THE CHANGE

By the time you reach the end of the thirtieth day of the programme, watch out for signs your body is giving you. Our body talks to us. Sometimes we just don't listen and hence we don't heal. There are signs indicating a change in your condition. The change isn't going to be major because it's only been four weeks, but is demonstrated in some of the following ways:

- On some days, you wake up a little fresher.
- On some days, your moods are better.
- The bloating and discomfort you felt in the first ten to fifteen days have begun to disappear. This means your gut has begun healing.
- If you needed to lose weight, you have lost some without doing heavy exercise.

On this programme, the body and mind reach a balanced state. Those who didn't need to lose weight, a couple of kilos will go—it was the bloating and toxins—and the rest will stay. Over time, warriors who are underweight will start gaining healthier weight. While excess toxins will get released, if you're not carrying excess weight, then you will not lose any unless you specifically try to by reducing how much you eat.

Gratitude is important

If you only complain and fail to be grateful for any improvements, it can slow down the process of healing. I have seen the perspective of gratitude being the difference in rates of healing in my patients with the same autoimmune condition and similar case history, age group and gender. Yogic breathing will help you incorporate a sense of gratitude.

Change is good but it also causes upheaval; embrace it

It's like shifting to a new house. For a few days your life will be disrupted. Your sleep quality will be poor in the new place, and you will be living out of unpacked boxes cluttered around the house. But that doesn't mean you run away from your beautiful new home. In the same manner, don't run away from your new normal.

Most importantly, be patient with yourself

We have a sixth sense that intuitively tells us whether we're healing or not. When we look for the positive signs, we start healing. When we heal, the cells of our body are more receptive to healing. So, appreciate beautiful music, the flavours of your food and the way the sheets caress your skin at night. This heightened sense of awareness starts helping us notice the things that we need to be grateful for.

You have embarked upon a healing journey that only the brave can do. No one will believe in you except yourself. Many of my patients come from families of doctors and they defy their parents to do my programme. In fact, a large number of my patients are doctors themselves. It's said that if you want to see change, change what's inside. That's what we're doing with clean eating, nutrition and pranayama.

This programme changes the way we think, feel and experience. The same things that were irritating and frustrating before now begin to feel trivial. Be receptive to experience these emotions. It takes years for many of us to let go of the pent-up emotions that triggered the disease. But awakening to it and walking towards this path begins now. Immerse yourself in this beautiful inner change.

Dr S.M. Sredevi, forty-four, is a gynaecologist from Coimbatore. After being diagnosed with RA, she signed up with me for treatment despite being a medical doctor herself. 'I followed the diet and exercise routine regularly but didn't give importance to sleep and rest,' she admits. 'I was undergoing a lot of stress in my personal life and had very little time to spend with my family because of work. I was the only gynaecologist in my area and was starting to feel burnt out.' Sredevi lost her father just before she was about to open her new nursing home but had to continue working because she was in a lot of debt. 'I have now started saying to myself that it's okay to take a break and rest,' she tells me. If a medical doctor can appreciate the importance of this protocol, so can you.

19
WORKING WITH YOUR DOCTOR

When I initially quit my medications and began holistic healing, I had a lot of anger against my rheumatologist. But today, I work with doctors to help their patients. Some specialists refer patients to me, some of whom are their family members. That's because medical science currently doesn't have a cure for autoimmune diseases. It's up to us to find a path to manage the illness.

Some warriors fear going back to their rheumatologist after they have healed. What if they lambast you for all the nutrition changes you have made, the supplements you are having? Keep in mind that rheumatologists do not specialize in nutrition. They are trained in medicine. If your rheumatologist sees your reports as clinically positive, they will start reducing your medications on their own. The key is to be on this healing protocol and keep medications to the lowest level so that your organs are protected, and your quality of life is high.

More than the rheumatologist, we need orthopaedics, yoga therapists and physiotherapists. Many warriors, including me, have damaged joints, so having a support system with these three specialties is important to continue healing and preventing future overload of toxic medications. As a yoga therapist, I know that the science of yoga also believes in combining the mind and body for healing and hence ventures into the intangible areas. Our brain is 10 per cent conscious and 90 per cent subconscious. Medical science knows about our conscious brain and how it directs the body. Yoga delves into the areas of the 90 per cent—the subconscious. An asana isn't just exercise; it also connects your body to your mind. It's not reactive like medical science but, rather, therapeutic.

Dr Jawahar Panjwani is a senior orthopaedic surgeon from Mumbai who has been doing joint replacement surgeries for autoimmune warriors. 'Joint replacement should only be an option when non-operative treatments don't provide substantial and sustained relief from pain, and daily activities become a challenge,' he says. In his view, exercise is paramount for mobility. 'Exercise has tremendous benefit in preserving mobility and enhancing muscle strength and bone density. It also gives a psychological boost because a good training session causes an abundant release of endorphins, which aids pain relief.'

When I first met Dr Panjwani and showed him my scans, he couldn't believe that they were mine. That was because I wasn't exhibiting any impact of the joint damage he saw in the scan. He told me that I had full movement and yet clinically it didn't correlate to what was in the scans. Medical science has limited belief in the ability of the mind and body to heal themselves. That's why people like me who have healed their autoimmune disease are called medical marvels—not because we have done anything special but because the perspective of medical science is based on reactivity.

Unfortunately, when we're ravaged by the multidimensional symptoms of autoimmune conditions, this reactive approach of medical science overloads us with medications, interventions

WORKING WITH YOUR DOCTOR

and procedures because we're not going to the root cause. Step back from that reactive mindset. Remember, an overreactive immune system was what led to this disease in the first place. Breathe deeply and start believing that you can heal. Then follow the programme as given in this book.

The case studies here are all real. If it has worked for them, it will work for you too. Then, work with your doctor from that perspective. However, if you believe in your doctor, follow him—but not without taking responsibility for yourself to follow the path of holistic nutrition to nurture yourself. Your quality of life depends only on you and your decisions.

20
WEIRD THINGS FOR SELF-HEALING

I was a certified nutritional therapist, but not yet a certified mental health therapist when I began treating others. I just went with my gut, asking myself, 'What will help me release my pent-up negative energy?' I devised my own ways, which I then shared with my patients. It helped them as well. I am listing some things I did during the healing process. While some of them may feel weird to you, don't judge—just try them. Once you get over your own inhibitions, you will start feeling free and light.

Just before sleeping, make loud sounds

Sigh loudly, like you're getting relief from pain. Say something like '*Aaaaaaaaaaaaaahhhhhhh …*' Fade out softly, not abruptly. Do it a few times. Doing this before you sleep releases your pent-up energy, frustration, pain and inflammation.

Shut the world out

Some days, I pull down the blinds or sit with my headphones by the sea or on my terrace. You can go to a nearby park with your headphones and shut the world out by playing healing music and being at one with whichever part of nature is accessible to you. It could be the sky if you have terrace access, some grass if you have a park nearby or the water if you live in a city near the sea or a river. Being alone in your own energy with nature helps you relax, recover and restore.

When in doubt, breathe

It's normal to feel overwhelmed, anxious, displaced and frustrated during this journey of healing. Whenever that happens, just put on some healing music and breathe deeply. I know it sounds impossible to do that when you are so wound up, but even a couple of minutes of deep breathing will start reducing your anxiety. If you give your mind and body the nurturing of slow and calm breathing, it will slowly calm down, lowering your anxiety and inflammation levels.

Make a list

We want to do so many things but because of chronic fatigue, we don't end up doing them. Make a list of things to do on the days you feel good. Keep adding to that list on the days you don't. When the good days increase, go to that list and start ticking them off. It could be a meal in a restaurant, watching a play, meeting friends, travelling—whatever is on your list, start implementing it as you get better. These matter because they make you feel free and normal.

Put yourself first

Choosing yourself means being kind not just to yourself but also to those you love. It also helps you heal faster. Life is all about choices. Choose you.

Get physical therapy

This need not be with a physical therapist, although that would be good too. It could be a restorative yoga class, or a simple foot massage. The soles of our feet have pressure points that help reduce pain. It will help you more than pain medicine. If your movement is restricted, get an expert to move your body and joints to increase circulation. When the circulation increases, you will see a reduction in fatigue, pain and bloating. Physical therapy could also be in the form of going to an acupuncture specialist to find relief. Physically getting relief through any form of therapy will help you move further towards your goal of healing.

Believe

Our beliefs have an overwhelming impact on our reality. When we have faith in a higher power, we believe that someone up there has our back. Similarly, when we believe in our ability to achieve something, our brain releases neurotransmitters such as dopamine, which increases our motivation and confidence. Negative thoughts can trap you in a vicious cycle of negativity, which will prevent your progress. Negativity can trigger stress responses to hinder healing. Believe that you can heal, and you will.

Join a class

It could be art or music therapy, maybe wine appreciation or perhaps Tai Chi. You will meet new people, experience new energy and learn new things. If the mind is diverted towards learning something new, we stop focusing on our disease symptoms. Find a class that you are interested in and physically capable of doing. If you feel physically incapable of joining a class, join an online class. This helps.

MANIFESTATION AND SELF-AFFIRMATION

'Manifestation' means to turn an idea into reality. If you visualize yourself being fine, science says that it *actually* makes you feel better. It has worked for me personally, especially when I felt low or down and out. During such times, I just lie down, close my eyes and start manifesting. These manifestations then turn into affirmations. A simple way to begin is by writing down your desired manifestations a couple of times a day. These repetitions through the day are believed to reinforce your intention and signal to the universe to make it happen.

In reality, it just makes you believe and gives you confidence that you can move forward. At a time when we're in pain and most medical professionals have told us there is no cure, this gives us confidence that we can still heal. It gives us hope, which is important because our mind needs hope to have the strength to believe. The success of self-affirmation is attributed to its ability to broaden a person's overall perspective and reduce the effect of negative emotions.[1]

Whenever I take a healing group class, I often end the class with the affirmations listed below. I sometimes say them out loud just before going to sleep. I'm lucky I have a spouse who sleeps soundly so he doesn't wake up and look at me weirdly. But he knows I do all this. These things have helped me and other warriors I take in group sessions; they could help you too. Or you could make your own list of manifestations as long as the words used in the manifestations are positive.

- I am physically and mentally agile.

- I have unlimited energy.
- Today, I nurture my body and mind to heal.
- I choose to be happy and content.
- I wake up energetic and motivated every day and look forward to making this day meaningful.
- My vascular system is relaxed and calm.
- My mind and body are relaxed and calm.
- I am independent and self-sufficient.
- I am healing and strengthening every day.
- Today was a great day for me.
- I am grateful for nurturing myself.
- I am grateful that the universe has my back.

21

COPING TECHNIQUES FOR CAREGIVERS

Often, loved ones and caregivers of autoimmune warriors are clueless about where to start. They want to help but they don't know where or how to begin. They're confused because even after the best treatments from the top doctors, their loved one isn't feeling better. Every day, caregivers see the person they love struggle to get up and do daily tasks. Depression and anxiety are common companions of autoimmune conditions, and this can lead to relationship breakdowns if the caregiver isn't able to understand what is going through the warrior's mind and body. It can also be extremely frustrating because they don't want the relationship to suffer but they feel like they're not getting through because the warrior has created a wall around themselves.

After a diagnosis of MS, a woman is six times more likely to be separated or divorced than a man, according to a study that examined gender roles in 'partner abandonment'. But the longer the marriage, the more likely the partner would stay. The study also found that the longer the marriage the more likely it would remain intact.[1] The most unfortunate part of the study for me was the headline: 'Men leave: separation and divorce far more common when the wife is the patient'. However, with many of the warriors I have treated, the presence of the spouse has only enhanced their healing. This happens when the caregiver or spouse begins taking a keen interest in the recovery of their loved one.

Most autoimmune warriors live with feelings of inadequacy and are unable to contribute to a fulfilling relationship. They are struggling at so many levels that they're unable to communicate their feelings to their caregivers. They become susceptible to other diseases as well, making it extremely complicated for the caregiver to help them. New research reveals that the symptoms of depression, stress, anxiety and anger seen in patients with RA were linked to atherosclerosis, which is a build-up of fatty deposits in the arteries that contributes to cardiovascular disease. The study was published in *Arthritis Care & Research*, a journal of the American College of Rheumatology. It suggests that screening and treatment of psychosocial symptoms may curb the cardiovascular disease.[2]

So as a caregiver, the first thing you need to do is to look after yourself well so that you're able to look after your loved one. If you neglect your mental health, you can start feeling emotionally overwhelmed—and physical illness soon follows. When you commit to a healthy lifestyle yourself, you are in a better position to encourage your loved ones to do the same. You can adapt to the nutrition and food protocol in this book so that the same food is on the table for the entire family. This way, the warrior doesn't feel isolated during their meals. The food recommendations are healthy and suitable for most people. It will help your health too and enable you in helping your loved one. Here are a few thing to keep in mind:

Don't be judgemental

Warriors may not feel like eating or waking up in the morning. They might be listless and not feel like doing even simple tasks. This is because of chronic fatigue. In many cases, this is seen as laziness, even by their caregiver. This is insensitive and can lead to the warrior becoming even more demotivated. The holistic nutritional plan will start working in three weeks' time to improve their energy and mood. Till that happens, don't judge how much they rest or sleep and their continued listlessness. Sit with them and encourage them.

If you love them, let them sleep

Sleep is essential to repair ourselves. Autoimmune warriors need more sleep because they need repair work at every level. Encouraging them to get into bed early and letting them sleep till late in the morning—which is the most healing time for them—can drastically accelerate the healing process. If the warrior resists sleep, remind them gently that if they sleep, they will get healthier.

You can consult the results of scientific research that I've referred to in this book to explain the positive impact of sleep on gut repair, inflammation and flare-ups. They want to get better and that is also what you want. So, ask if they won't do it for themselves, will they do it for you? At this stage, emotional frailty is high, so an emotional appeal from the caregiver may be what's needed for the warrior to agree to rest and sleep more.

Help them organize their schedule

Even for healthy people, it's difficult in the first couple of weeks to adapt to a new schedule or way of doing things. For warriors, it's even tougher. They feel overwhelmed and disorganized. Make a schedule as per my programme so that it's simpler for them to follow. Put printouts on the fridge so that they're always reminded of their plan for the day. If you have someone else cooking your meals, get them to follow the recipes provided in this book. If not, cook them yourself so that your loved one doesn't get tired by preparing their own meals. Remember to encourage and support them by keeping what *they* need to eat on the table. Don't offer a bite of what you're eating—that maybe they like too—because you feel bad for them. Such acts of 'pity' will derail their nutritional plan.

Create a meditation or relaxation playlist for them

In line with my recommendations, they can just play healing music and start doing their breathing exercises instead of searching for the right music every time.

Open the home energy for them

Clutter around the house increases the chances of the warrior to get hurt or fall because their balance is poor. So tidy up around the house as much as possible. To reduce any chance of their falling in the bathroom, put antiskid mats and add handles to the wall for support. Increase the seat height of the bed, chairs and sofa to twenty inches from the floor as that is ideal for the lower back and knees to feel supported and for the joints to stay protected.

Increase oxygen

Oxygen is a big healer for autoimmune warriors, so place twenty-four-hour oxygen emitting indoor plants around the house. This is especially important in the areas where they do their breathing exercises. Easily available plants for the home include Areca palm, peace lily, snake plant, aloe vera and money plant.

Take them out

Your loved one will not feel like dressing up and stepping out because they're feeling so low. But being in fresh air and sunlight will help their healing. You could take them on a drive to a scenic place such as a garden, the banks of a river or the seaside. This will help them be in nature.

Set dates with them

If the warrior is a significant other, you could plan a date with them. As their energy increases, plan frequent romantic moments. Take them to a restaurant or to a park with a picnic hamper. Small surprises, such as a treat made with permitted ingredients to remind them that you love them, would go a long way in making the warrior happier.

However, be prepared for outbursts. Even if you're doing your best, accept that the warrior may have an emotional breakdown. They may not be looking for solutions but just unconditional emotional support. Don't lecture them or advise them at such times. Just be with them and support them without giving your opinion. Understand that they're going through something that you may never be able to understand, no matter how much you love them. This can sound demoralizing but remember: even medical science doesn't understand autoimmune diseases and hence there is no cure. So don't feel bad, guilty or demotivated. Your unconditional support will help them recover faster.

22

COPING TECHNIQUES FOR THE WARRIOR

'Sorry I am late. I sat on my bed in a towel for an hour staring at the wall after a bath.'

This statement resonates with so many warriors! Fatigue can make even a bath seem exhausting for a warrior, as many of us have experienced. This stems from our poor energy levels, which makes it difficult to even do everyday tasks. Every little thing takes more time, and the brain fog stops us from moving forward. So it is really important to do the following:

Rest, rest, rest

If you can't rest for long because of your work, take mini breaks. If you can't sleep in till late in the morning, then take a twenty-minute mid-morning nap with music in the background and your phone in another room. Make the room dark so that you feel like you're in a quiet, soothing place. In fact, take three fifteen-minute naps during a working day: one mid-morning, one after lunch and one at 5 p.m. This will drastically reduce chronic fatigue and increase your energy levels. It may seem impossible to you to take these naps at work but you'll be surprised that nobody misses you for such short gaps. Make it happen.

Plan in advance

You will have spurts of energy and clarity. Use those moments to plan your tasks and food. Plan meals and supplements for a week in advance.

Make your life as predictable as possible

This will help you to mechanically follow your routine until your brain fog lifts. Repetitive tasks will not be so boring in your condition because your ability to think creatively is compromised. Continuously doing what needs to be done will begin the miracle of your restoration to health.

It's okay to have an outburst

Autoimmune conditions are related to suppression, so sometimes, crying or expressing negative emotions and frustrations can be a good thing. Don't hold yourself back if you really need to do this. But don't make such outbursts a habit.

Remember that your caregiver can't read your mind

Help them understand your emotions by having conversations. Try to talk through what is bothering you even if it may seem trivial to them. It will help you release it from your system and will reduce their frustrations too. Expressing and releasing negative emotions will aid your journey of healing.

The ability of the human body to repair itself is scientifically proven. Believe it

When you start to despair and wonder why you are suffering so much, try to remember that if you focus on the holistic nutritional treatment, you will reach a stage where your symptoms are going to start disappearing. Keep reminding yourself of your body's ability to heal itself and have faith in it. Always remember that nothing is permanent. Whatever you're going through today, it this too shall pass.

23
DOUSING FLARE-UPS

Once you get to your new normal, you will feel highly energetic and mentally more positive especially because your clinical markers will almost be within normal range. However, do remember that to stay healed for the rest of your life, you will need to be tuned in to the signs your body is giving you. That way you will know when a flare-up is coming. When that happens, carrying out the necessary steps will help you dodge the flare-up. Understanding why a flare-up gets triggered and how you can douse the fire is important for leading a steadily healthy life. Here are a few points to bear in mind:

Flare-up triggers

The most common flare-up triggers are emotional. If you have experienced an emotionally distressing situation, be mindful of following the tenets of the programme—nutrition, pranayama and yoga—so that your emotional immunity remains stable. Food can be a trigger—usually sour items. Other flare-ups can result from skipping pranayama or not getting adequate sleep. Once you have identified your triggers, it's easy to plug the holes and reverse a flare-up within forty-eight hours.

Whatever the trigger, the first thing you need to do is get complete rest

You need a reboot. Unplug your devices, switch off your phone and listen to music. You could even read a book or watch a funny movie.

Go back to Phase 1

In Phase 1, there are only gut-pacifying and anti-inflammatory foods and pranayama but no exercise. When you experience a flare-up, stop exercise and follow the diet and breathwork of Phase 1. This will help calm your emotional immunity and give your body the rest it needs to release emotional fatigue.

The power of humour

If you do choose to watch a funny movie, make sure it really is laugh-out-loud funny and not a somewhat amusing family drama. The vascular system, also known as the circulatory system, is made up of vessels which carry blood and lymph through the body, and laughter has a positive impact on our vascular function.[1] Autoimmune conditions impact this system, causing multidimensional symptoms throughout the body. The moment we experience laughter, the vascular system starts reducing inflammation in the body. And hence, laughter becomes a key factor in reducing the flare-up within a day or two.

Try to sleep for nine hours at night

Do include the very restful and healing morning sleep, wake up late. Then nap for half an hour in the afternoon. At this time, your body is going through a lot of oxidative stress.

Up your intake of vitamin C

Since most autoimmune conditions are connective-tissue disorders, increasing your intake of vitamin C will enable your body to start producing more collagen, thus reducing inflammation levels. While the regular daily intake prescribed in my programme is 500 mg three times a day after meals, during a flare-up this should be doubled for three to seven days. Therefore, you need to take 1 g of vitamin C after every meal three times a day on those days. This doesn't apply to those with a kidney-related autoimmune condition. Ensure to reduce doses for children proportionately, as instructed earlier.

24
MOVING FORWARD

The following food items will continue to not be allowed for one year: spinach, kale, sour items, bell peppers, eggplant, lentils and pulses, red meat, tea, coffee, milk, milk products, wheat, white flour and other forms of gluten. Okra and bitter gourd can be consumed once in ten days after one year. Watch out for adverse gut reactions. If that happens, eliminate them from your diet.

Remember your four pillars:

- elimination diet
- nutritional supplements
- breathwork and yoga
- rest and sleep

These make your foundation strong.

Choose your poison to be added back

Whether it takes twelve months or twenty-four, from the day you are symptomatically and clinically negative, you can choose a food that you were not allowed to have and add it to the allowed list. Except for sour items, you can choose any one food and have it once a week—but not more than that. For example, if you love cheese, you can have small quantities once a week as long as your symptoms are completely gone.

It's okay to continue some medications

For some warriors, nutritional healing sometimes doesn't manage to reduce all symptoms. They choose to combine holistic healing with medications. Decide what combination works best for you. Whatever you decide, without holistic nutrition, your quality of life is going to be poor. But if the medications are not extremely toxic, their side effects are usually taken care of by the nutrition, yoga and pranayama plan.

For example, if you have dry eyes, get a good lubricant eyedrop prescribed. Some eyedrops come with nutrients like N-acetylcarnosine (NAC). As an antioxidant, NAC is able to combat effects of oxidative stress. It can stop the lens from becoming cloudy and improve vision. Some medications have severe side effects. They can't manage your condition nor give you a better quality of life.

When you follow your new normal protocol, your reports will be clinically better. This is scientific evidence that your body is healing. Consistently continue with the four pillars even after being clinically negative. You can adjust supplements as per vitamin reports. An autoimmune patient can't be treated just by suppressing localized symptoms. Pain, anxiety, gut health and chronic fatigue are all linked to a poor quality of life. Addressing everything *together* is what heals the immune system.

PART 5

Food heals. Emotions heal. And the joy of life returns.

25
DAYS LIKE THIS

'I feel my RA was triggered by a combination of pregnancy, Covid, past trauma, taking tums (antacid) during pregnancy and a C-section. Four years before the onset of RA, my heart was broken when an engagement to be married didn't work out, in a very traumatic way. I also experienced major trauma as a child. I felt depressed as soon as I was diagnosed and during flare-ups, I went on a light antidepressant right away to take the edge off because I was three months postpartum when diagnosed.

'I never thought it was incurable. I knew it was reversible and that's why I kept searching until I found Rachna! I didn't try anything before I went to her because I refused to go on methotrexate and as soon as I was diagnosed, I went down a rabbithole until I found her online one night and I knew this was the answer. Breathwork and music (our favourite—Van Morrison!) help a lot. Also knowing that a flare-up will pass when having a flare-up and that I am not alone.

'But frankly, when I initially began, I didn't believe that just eating and breathing right would do the trick. I was very fearful. The cleanse/detox made a huge difference and the breathwork helped immensely! Right away! Within weeks, I began seeing major changes and within a month, the inflammation levels in my blood work were back to normal levels.

'Before I met Rachna, I used to be depressed, overweight/inflamed, and experiencing postpartum symptoms, extreme pain in big muscles and joints. I could barely sit up or get off the ground. But after her treatment I began to feel empowered, have appreciation for my body, I feel healthy, active, fewer flare-ups and bearable and manageable pain, I feel great in my own skin! And most importantly, I am hopeful and determined! Follow the plan Rachna gives you to the tee at first (for the first three months at least!) and it will pay off later!

'I am a mom to a one-and-a-half-year-old wild, brilliant and sweet boy! I practice acupuncture, pilates and skincare. I am a warrior of love and light. I am passionate about music, art, connection, the ocean, sunshine and dancing! I plan to help my patients and others with chronic pain and autoimmune disease that I know by being the example and helping them walk down their own healing path. I recommend Rachna to anyone that comes my way looking for help and who is struggling!'

—*Michele LaVire, 42, Vail, Colorado.*

I miss the email interactions I used to have with Michele. Because of our time zones not matching, we never did video sessions. But it was the unlimited email-based support, the charts and her following everything to the tee that made a huge impact on her healing journey. The most delightful part was that during the course of my treatment, she wanted to go for a Van Morrison concert. Just after her twenty-one-day cleanse, she emailed me: 'Next week we're going out of town to see Van Morrison so please let me know what to eat when I travel :).' I couldn't refuse so I sent her the travel dos and don'ts in exchange for pictures and videos of the concert! Sitting in Mumbai, she helped me enjoy Van Morrison live.

DAYS LIKE THIS

This song of his reflects how we feel when we're healed.

When you don't need to worry there'll be days like this
When no one's in a hurry there'll be days like this [...]
Oh my mama told me there'll be days like this
When all the parts of the puzzle start to look like they fit it
Then I must remember there'll be days like this
There'll be days like this

—'Days Like This', *Van Morrison*

100 RECIPES

To eat delicious food is divine.

You can follow the prescribed meal plans by using these easy recipes. Keep in mind that these recipes are modified with only the permitted ingredients in this programme. You may see many of your favourite dishes listed, but the original preparation might not be allowed. Don't use any of recipes for the dish from the internet or a cookbook—only follow these modified recipes for your favourite dishes.

To recap some of the earlier advice about food and cooking:

- *No packet or powdered masala.* This is because when they're powdered, spices are in a concentrated form, which can irritate the lining of the gut. Packet masalas also have high levels of toxins.
- *Whole spices are good.* Do add whole spices as per your taste, but not too much. Temper your food with mild flavours.
- *Eat three meals and two snacks every day.* Without continuous nourishment, your chronic fatigue will not lift.
- *Don't skip on protein.* After the first phase, you need to eat eggs, chicken breast, oily fish or tofu as required. For those who don't eat any of these, you can increase your vegan protein in the form of almond milk, adding a tablespoon of protein powder (see p. 213) and dates syrup (see p. 210) at least once or twice a day. Lack of protein will cause muscle fatigue and pain. So don't skimp on daily protein levels.

- *Include foods high in potassium and magnesium daily.* Hypokalemia is when the amount of potassium in your blood is too low.[1] Low magnesium levels also lead to low potassium and that can increase muscle cramps, spasms and twitches and also be a cause of low pulse rate, weakness, fatigue and hypertension. Since many potassium-rich foods—such as banana, spinach, peanuts, cashews and tomatoes—are not allowed, make sure you include other nutrient-rich foods such as broccoli, potatoes, avocados, almonds and quinoa on a regular basis. This doesn't apply to those with kidney-related autoimmune conditions.

- *Give yourself time to adapt.* This kind of eating is new to you. At first, your mind and body are going to resist. You will start adapting to this new clean eating within a couple of weeks.

1. Aloe vera juice

Ingredients

6-inch medium broad aloe vera leaf
300 ml drinking/purified water

Method

- In a blender, add 100 ml water and a small cut of aloe vera leaf; mix well.
- Next, add 200 ml water to make the juice.
- Store in the fridge and mix 1 tablespoon daily in your morning water. Make it fresh weekly. If you don't have an aloe vera plant, look for readymade aloe vera juice that doesn't contain any citrus or additives.

2. Poha

Ingredients

1 cup thick poha
1 tbsp rice bran oil
1 tsp mustard seeds
1 tsp cumin seeds
8–10 curry leaves, fresh or air dried
½ tsp ground organic turmeric

1–2 green chillies
1–2 cloves of garlic, minced
1 large onion, finely chopped
1 medium sized potato, peeled and chopped
Himalayan or sea salt to taste
½ cup coriander leaves, washed and chopped

Method

- Rinse poha in a colander or sieve, drain and keep aside.
- Heat oil in a pan over high heat. Add the mustard seeds. Let the mustard seeds pop. Then lower the heat, add cumin seeds, curry leaves, green chillies, turmeric and stir.
- Add the onions, mix well and cook covered for a couple of minutes on medium heat as they start to soften.
- Stir in the potatoes and salt. Cook covered till the potatoes are done.
- Add the poha and mix. Cook covered on low heat for 5 more minutes or till the poha is done.
- Garnish with coriander and serve hot.

3. Quinoa upma with permitted vegetables

Ingredients

200 gm quinoa, boiled
1 medium-sized onion, finely chopped
1 tbsp rice bran oil
1–2 cloves of garlic, minced
4–5 curry leaves
1 tsp mustard seeds

½ tsp cumin seeds
½ cup of three permitted vegetables, finely chopped
½ cup water
A pinch of organic turmeric powder
Salt and pepper to taste

Method

- Boil quinoa till it's very soft and keep aside.
- In a pan, add 1 tablespoon rice bran oil and stir-fry onions, garlic, curry leaves, mustard seeds and cumin seeds.
- Add the chopped vegetables and stir-fry for 2 minutes.
- Add ½ cup water, turmeric, black pepper and salt.
- Slowly add the boiled quinoa and simmer for 7–10 minutes. Add water for semi-liquid consistency if required. Simmer for 5–7 minutes more. Switch off and serve warm.

4. Brown rice upma with permitted vegetables

Ingredients

3–4 tbsp brown rice flour (for one serving)
1–2 cloves of garlic, minced
1 tbsp rice bran oil
1 medium-sized onion, finely chopped
4–5 curry leaves
1 tsp mustard seeds
½ tsp cumin seeds
A total of ½ cup of three permitted vegetables, finely chopped
1 cup water—half for dissolving flour and half for cooking
A pinch of organic turmeric powder

Salt and pepper to taste

Method

- Dissolve 3 tablespoons of brown rice flour in water till it has a batter consistency. Ensure that there are no lumps. Keep aside.
- In a pan, add 1 tablespoon rice bran oil, then stir-fry the onions, garlic, curry leaves, mustard seeds, cumin seeds, then add the chopped vegetables and stir-fry for 2 minutes.
- Add ½ cup water, turmeric, black pepper and salt.
- Slowly add the dissolved rice flour into the vegetables and simmer for 7–10 minutes. Add water for semi-liquid consistency if required. Simmer for 5–7 minutes. Switch off the heat and serve warm.

5. Brown rice porridge

Ingredients

200 ml almond milk
50 ml water
2 tbsp brown rice flour
1 tbsp dates syrup (see p. 210)

Method

- Add the almond milk in a pan and simmer.
- Dissolve the rice flour in approximately 50 ml water, or till you get a batter-like consistency. Ensure that there are no lumps.
- Slowly add the rice porridge to the almond milk and simmer for 2–3 minutes. Switch off the heat.

- Add dates syrup for sweetness. This makes a very nourishing pick-me-up drink!

6. Dosa

Ingredients

1 cup quinoa, parboiled
1 cup white rice, parboiled
1 tsp cumin seeds
Dried red chillies (optional)
1 cup water
2-inch piece of bottle gourd, peeled
1 medium-sized onion, finely chopped
4–5 curry leaves
A bunch of washed coriander leaves, finely chopped
1 tsp baking soda
Rice bran oil
Salt and pepper to taste

Method

- Soak the parboiled rice and quinoa with baking soda for three hours. Drain and mix in cumin seeds, dried red chillies and a cup of water. Grind the mixture to a very slightly coarse paste.
- Grate the bottle gourd. A 2-inch piece should make ½ cup grated bottle gourd. If the bottle gourd is very ripe, remove the seeds and then grate it.
- Add the grated bottle gourd to the ground rice batter along with the onion, curry leaves and coriander leaves. Add in salt and pepper as per taste.

- Make the batter thin so that the dosas crisp up nicely on the griddle. Add water if required and adjust the batter to desired consistency.
- Heat a dosa pan over medium heat until it is hot.
- Add the rice bran oil and then add half a cup of dosa batter and spread it evenly on the pan. Since the batter is thin, you can't swirl the dosa, so just use a ladle to spread it out.
- Cook the dosa for 1 minute on each side. Repeat with the remaining batter, ensuring to mix the batter well each time.

7. Poha cutlets

Ingredients

1 cup thick poha
1 large potato, mashed
1 small carrot, grated
5 French beans, finely chopped
1 onion, finely chopped
15–20 coriander leaves, washed and chopped
½ tsp ginger-garlic paste (fresh)
¼ tsp turmeric
¼ tsp organic red chilli powder (optional)
½ tsp homemade garam masala
½ tsp dry mango powder
1 tsp white sesame seeds
Salt to taste
3 tbsp oil

Method

- Rinse the poha twice and soak it in enough water so that it just about covers it. Leave it for 3–4 minutes, then drain the water.
- Add all the vegetables and spices. Mix well and shape into small cutlets.
- Heat a granite or ceramic pan and add oil. When hot, place the cutlets on the pan. Cook on low to medium heat. They are ready when golden-brown and crisp on both sides.
- Serve with mint chutney.

8. Brown rice salted pancake

Ingredients

1 cup brown rice flour
75 ml water
1 medium-sized onion, finely chopped
Fresh coriander/parsley leaves, washed and chopped
1 green chilli, optional
A pinch of carom seeds
Salt and pepper to taste
A pinch of organic turmeric powder
Water for batter consistency
1 tbsp rice bran oil

Method

- Dissolve brown rice flour in 75 ml water, or till you get a batter-like consistency.

- Add onions, coriander or parsley, chopped green chilli, a pinch of carom seeds, salt, pepper and turmeric. Mix well and add water to make it into a smooth batter consistency.
- In a granite saucepan, add 1 tablespoon of rice bran oil. Add all the ingredients apart from the flour and stir-fry for 2–3 minutes. Reduce the flame and then add the rice flour, spreading it evenly. Flip to make both sides crispy and golden-brown.
- Serve with coriander or pesto chutney.

9. Idli without lentils

Ingredients

    1 cup brown rice flour
    2 cups rice flour, coarsely ground
    1 cup bottle gourd, grated
    1 carrot, grated
    75–100 ml water
    Fresh coriander leaves, washed, chopped
    1 tsp fenugreek seeds, powdered
    Salt and pepper to taste

Method

- In a pan, add the white and brown rice flour, grated bottle gourd and carrots, coriander leaves, fenugreek seeds powder, salt and pepper to taste and water and make into a paste. Cover and keep for 1 hour.
- Next, add the batter into an idli steamer and steam for 10–15 minutes.
- Serve with coriander chutney.

10. White rice vermicelli

Ingredients

75 gm white rice vermicelli (check the packet's ingredients; it should only contain rice, water and salt. Easily available in Japanese vermicelli brands.)

1 tbsp rice bran oil

1 medium-sized onion, finely chopped

1 tsp mustard seeds

4 curry leaves

½ tsp turmeric

A pinch of black pepper

Salt to taste

Coriander leaves, washed and chopped

Method

- In a cast iron or ceramic pan, heat 1 tablespoon rice bran oil on medium heat, add onions, mustard seeds and curry leaves and cook till they crackle. Keep the tadka aside.
- In a steel pan, add 1 litre water and bring to a boil. Add the vermicelli and boil till it is soft. Drain the water and wash the vermicelli.
- In a pan on medium flame, add the seasoning/tadka with the vermicelli, add turmeric, pepper, chopped coriander, mix well and switch off the heat.

11. Vegan omelette

Ingredients

2–3 tbsp white or brown rice flour

1 tbsp rice bran oil
½ onion, chopped
¼ carrot, grated (optional)
1 tbsp peas
Fresh coriander leaves, well washed, finely chopped
2 garlic cloves, minced
Salt and black pepper to taste
1 green chilli, finely chopped (optional)
Vegan cheese as per taste (see p. 208)

Method

- Dissolve the rice flour in water so that it becomes a thin but smooth paste. Keep aside for 30 minutes and then check the consistency. If it is too thick, add more water.
- In a granite saucepan, add 1 tablespoon of rice bran oil on medium heat. Add all the ingredients (except the flour batter) and stir-fry for 2–3 minutes. Reduce the heat and then add the rice flour, spreading it evenly. Flip to make both sides crispy and golden-brown.
- Serve with coriander or pesto chutney.

12. Turmeric quinoa risotto

Ingredients

1 cup stir-fried vegetables (see p. 230)
½ cup quinoa, half boiled, kept aside
200 ml almond milk
A pinch of organic turmeric
1 tbsp almond butter
Salt and pepper to taste

Method

- Parboil the quinoa and keep aside.
- Stir-fry vegetables as per stir-fry recipe and keep aside.
- In a pan, add the almond milk, turmeric, black pepper, almond butter and the parboiled quinoa and let it simmer. When the quinoa is soft, add the stir-fry vegetables to this and simmer for a minute on low heat, and then switch it off. Serve hot/warm.

13. Turmeric white rice risotto

Ingredients

1 cup stir-fried vegetables (see p. 230)
200 ml almond milk
A pinch of organic turmeric
1 tbsp almond butter
Salt and pepper to taste
½ cup white rice, parboiled, kept aside

Method

- Stir-fry vegetables as per stir-fry recipe and keep aside.
- In a pan, add the almond milk, turmeric, almond butter, salt and black pepper and the parboiled rice and let it simmer.
- When the rice is soft, add the stir-fried vegetables and switch off the heat. Serve hot.

14. Buckwheat *(kuttu)* dosa

Ingredients

½ tbsp white rice

½ cup buckwheat (kuttu)
Coriander leaves
2 tbsp rice bran oil
1 tsp mustard seeds
1 green chilli, finely chopped
Salt to taste

Method

- Grind the rice along with the buckwheat to a fine powder and keep aside.
- Next, heat 1 tablespoon of oil in a frying pan and add the mustard seeds. When the seeds start to pop, add asafoetida and sauté over medium heat for a few seconds. Then, add the chopped green chillies and a cup of water, and mix well. Allow the mixture to cool down before gently pouring it into the rice-flour mixture.
- Blend the flour with the water slowly to create a smooth batter. Add salt. Adjust the amount of rice as needed to get the right batter consistency.
- Grease a ceramic pan with a few drops of oil and spread a small amount of the batter from the centre. Cook till both sides turn golden-brown. Serve hot with vegetables.

15. Rice pancake

Ingredients

4–5 tbsp white rice flour
½ tsp carom seeds

1 tbsp rice bran oil
Salt and pepper to taste

Method

- Dissolve the rice flour in water to make a batter-like consistency.
- Add the other ingredients to the batter.
- Heat a pan or griddle on medium heat. Add ½ cup batter and spread it evenly. Cook the pancake for a minute on each side. Repeat with the rest of the batter. Mix the batter well each time.

16. Potato pancakes

Ingredients

4–5 tbsp boiled mashed potatoes
½ tsp carom seeds
1 tbsp EVOO
2 garlic cloves, minced
Salt and pepper to taste
1 tbsp rice bran oil

Method

- Mix all the ingredients (except for the rice bran oil) to make a dough.
- Make into pancake shapes.
- Add rice bran oil to a pan and shallow fry till they're crispy on each side. Serve hot.

17. Almond-flour pancakes

Ingredients

1 large potato
1 medium onion
1 organic egg
2 tbsp fresh coriander leaves, chopped
Salt to taste
4 heaped tbsp almond flour
1 heaped tbsp psyllium husk
3–4 tbsp olive oil

Method

- Finely grate the potatoes and onion. Get rid of any excess water. Add in the egg, coriander leaves and salt. Mix well with the almond flour and psyllium husk to make into a batter. Add water to adjust the consistency.
- In a granite or ceramic pan, add the oil and 2 tablespoons of the batter, giving it a round shape. Cook till both sides are brown and crisp.
- Remove them from the pan and place on a kitchen towel to drain any extra oil.
- The pancakes can be served with 1 tablespoon of honey.

18. Coriander chutney

Ingredients

1 cup coriander leaves, washed and without stems
4 tbsp EVOO

20 raw almonds
3–4 garlic cloves, peeled
2–3 green chillies, chopped (optional)
1 tbsp mustard oil
1 tsp mustard seeds
5–6 curry leaves
1 tsp salt

Method

- Soak the coriander leaves with a teaspoon of salt dissolved in the water. Drain after five minutes and keep aside.
- Add EVOO to the raw almonds, coriander leaves, garlic and chillies, add water and blend. Keep aside.
- Heat mustard oil in a small steel or ceramic pan and add the mustard seeds and curry leaves. Cook on high flame for 3–4 minutes before switching off the heat.
- Add the blended mixture and salt and mix well with a spoon.

19. Red hummus dip

Ingredients

2 carrots, roasted
2 onions, chopped
3–4 garlic cloves
30 mamra almonds
1 green chilli (optional)
Salt to taste
4–5 tbsp EVOO
Drinking/purified water as per consistency required

Method

- Add all the ingredients in a blender, then add a small quantity of water and blend well. If you add too much water, the blending will not be smooth. You can add more water as per consistency required and mix well.

20. Coriander and pine nuts pesto

Ingredients

A bunch of well washed coriander leaves
3–4 garlic cloves
30–40 pine nuts
1 green chilli (optional)
Salt and pepper to taste
4–5 tbsp EVOO
Drinking/purified water as per consistency required

Method

- Add all the ingredients to a blender, then add a small quantity of water and blend well. If you add too much water, the blending will not be smooth. You can add more water as per consistency required and mix well.

21. Avocado dip

Ingredients

2 ripe avocados
¼ cup almond butter
2 tbsp fresh coriander, finely chopped

2 garlic cloves, roasted and crushed
4 tbsp EVOO + 1 tbsp to drizzle
½ tsp chilli flakes (optional)
Sea salt to taste

Method

- Add all the ingredients to a blender in this order: avocado, almond butter, coriander, garlic, olive oil, chilli flakes and salt. Blend till the dip is smooth and there are no lumps. You may have to stop the blending every 30 seconds to scrape down the sides of the bowl with a spoon and then restart.
- Transfer the dip into a large bowl. Refrigerate for at least 1 hour to allow the flavours to blend.
- Drizzle 1 tablespoon of EVOO on top of the dip before serving.

22. Creamy pumpkin dip

Ingredients

¾ cup pumpkin or bottle gourd, roasted
1 avocado
1 garlic clove, crushed
1 tsp wholegrain gluten-free mustard
½ tsp sea salt
Freshly ground black pepper to taste
2 tbsp water

Method

- Blend all the ingredients until smooth and creamy. Add more water if you like it thinner. Serve cold.

23. Mixed nutrients dip

Ingredients

2 garlic cloves
15–30 arugula leaves
12–15 freshly washed coriander leaves
2 garlic cloves
1 cup broccoli, chopped and sautéed
1 onion, chopped
½ avocado, mashed
4 tbsp EVOO
Salt to taste
Green chillies, chopped (optional)

Method

- In a blender, add garlic, arugula and coriander leaves and blend well.
- Next, add the vegetables, avocado, EVOO, salt and optional green chillies. Mix well.
- Serve as a dip or use to top pizzas and crackers.

24. Vegan almond cheese

Ingredients

1 cup whole raw unsalted almonds
500 ml hot water
500 ml + 50 ml cold water
3 tbsp EVOO
Salt as specified in steps
½ tsp mix of dried herbs like oregano, thyme, rosemary

A pinch of black pepper
2 garlic cloves, crushed

Method

- Boil water and switch off the heat. Soak the almonds in the boiling hot water for 20 minutes, then drain and rinse.
- Next, either rub the almonds with a towel or just use your fingers to peel the skin off. Soak the blanched almonds in cold water, cover and refrigerate and for twenty-four hours.
- The next day, drain and rinse the almonds well before adding them to a grinder with the EVOO, salt and 50 ml water. Blend until smooth.
- Scrape the mixture into a double-layered cheesecloth or a fine handkerchief.
- Add the dried herbs, pepper, ½ teaspoon of salt and crushed garlic and mix well. Gather the cloth tightly around the almond mixture and make a bag by using a rubber band to tie the top. Give the bag a few gentle squeezes to remove any liquid. Put the bundle in a metal sieve and let the water drain into a bowl below it. Put the sieve and the bowl in the refrigerator overnight. This helps the cheese become denser.
- After 12 hours, carefully peel off the cloth. The cheese will feel like a cake dough. If you like it fresh, you can eat it in this form as soft cheese.
- Add salt and pepper as per your taste.
- You could also gently shape it into a square baking dish and bake it at 150°C for 30–40 minutes. Baking makes the top firm while the inside will still be creamy. Salt, garlic, herbs and black pepper will make this cheese very tasty.

Note: Even though I wouldn't normally recommend soaking and removing the skin of almonds, vegan cheese is healthier than eating dairy, so we can take this liberty. Removing the skin before making almond cheese gives the cheese a smoother texture and a lighter colour that looks like regular cheese. On the other hand, you can make the cheese with the almond skin on if you prefer.

25. Dates syrup

Ingredients

20 dates, deseeded
Drinking/purified water as per consistency required

Method

- Soak the deseeded dates in warm water for 1 hour. Peel the top layer and then blend the soft dates with ½ cup water.
- Use a heavy duty blender because a hand blender can get stuck due to the density of the dates. Add more water if required for a syrupy consistency. When the dates syrup is blended to a smooth consistency, transfer to a glass container, cover and store in the refrigerator. You can store this for a week. You can enjoy it out of the jar as a dessert or mix 1 teaspoon in warm almond milk. It also goes well with any of the pancake recipes in this book.

26. Green tea masala

Ingredients

1 tbsp organic turmeric
10 cloves

10 cardamoms

5 sticks of cinnamon, cut into 2-inch pieces

5 pieces aniseed

1 tsp freshly ground pepper

1 tsp fennel

Method

- Add all the ingredients to a blender and dry grind them to a powder. Store in a glass jar in a cool place.
- You can mix ½ teaspoon of this powder into your daily afternoon green tea. If you like, make a larger batch of masala by increasing quantities of the ingredients proportionately. But store it only in a glass container, not plastic.

27. Rice milk

Ingredients

To boil the rice
1 cup rice
2 cups water

To make rice water
Drinking/purified water as given in recipe

For tempering (optional)
1 tsp cumin seeds
1 tsp mustard seeds
5–6 curry leaves
Salt and pepper to taste

Method

- Add the rice to a pressure cooker and cook till it's done. We use this method to preserve all the water-soluble nutrients.
- Blend 2 tablespoons of cooked rice and 3 tablespoons of water in a high-speed blender for around 20 seconds, then stop and check the consistency. Add ½ cup of water and blend again if required. Please remember that if you blend with a lot of water right from the start, it will not be smooth. You have to blend it a little first before adding small quantities of water to it. Ensure that there is enough water added so that it becomes thin and creamy. If you blend it till it's creamy, it won't require sieving. However, it's not good to have any sediment left in the milk, so blend well, then use a cheesecloth to filter out any remaining sediment.
- You can add a tempering of mustard seeds, cumin seeds, curry leaves, salt and pepper for a cooling drink that is perfect to ease heartburn.

28. Nourishing popsicles

Ingredients

1 fresh pomegranate, peeled and separated
1 tbsp chia seeds
10 mint leaves

Method

- Crush the pomegranate and chia seeds, add the mint leaves and make into a smoothie using a blender.
- Once the smoothie paste is made, dilute by adding more water. Put the mix into ice trays and freeze. You can use the same recipe for cucumber popsicles as well.

29. Almond milk thandai

Ingredients

200 ml almond milk
1 tbsp khus
1 tbsp pomegranate
1 tbsp chia seeds
2 green cardamoms, crushed
1 tsp dates syrup (see p. 210)

Method

- Blend 30 ml of the almond milk with all the other ingredients. It will form a thick, coarse paste. Add the remaining almond milk and blend again for two minutes.
- Refrigerate and serve chilled.

30. Warm almond milk protein drink

Ingredients

200 ml almond milk
1 tsp dates syrup (see p. 210)
1 tbsp protein powder (see below)

- In a pan, warm the almond milk but don't bring it to a boil.
- Add the other ingredients and mix well. Have this when you are feeling low on energy.

31. Protein powder

Ingredients

100 gm almonds

100 gm pistachios
100 gm chia seeds

Method

- Dry grind equal amounts of almonds, pistachios and chia seeds in a blender. Store the powder in a glass jar in the refrigerator. This is a perfect vegan protein powder that is high in iron too.
- Add to almond milk (see previous recipe), sprinkle on salads or just mix with organic honey and have it as a snack.

32. Mulled wine

Note: This is an alcoholic beverage. However, wine has proven anti-inflammatory properties because of the presence of resveratrol. Combined with the healing properties of the spices in this recipe, it becomes a wholesome drink with minimal alcohol. After the first thirty days of detox, you can have this twice a week if you like.

Ingredients

200 ml red wine
50 ml apple juice
1 tbsp honey
2–3 cardamom pods
1–2 cinnamon sticks
2 pieces of star anise

Method

- Add 200 ml wine to a large pot and allow it to simmer.

- Add all the other ingredients. Keep simmering to allow the spices to infuse into the wine.
- Serve warm. This drink has warming properties so it is best suited to winter evenings when the cold affects your joints.

33. Celery and broccoli soup

Ingredients

2 tbsp olive oil
½ onion, diced
1–2 fat garlic cloves, roughly chopped
2 cups celery, sliced thin (save some for garnishing)
3 florets broccoli, chopped
1 small potato, sliced into ½-inch thick rounds
Salt and pepper to taste
¼ cup fresh dill
½ cup fresh parsley
30 ml almond milk

Method

- Heat oil in a pan and add onions and stir.
- Now, add the garlic and stir for 1–2 minutes.
- Add chopped celery, broccoli, potatoes, salt and pepper, and top up with water to cover the vegetables. Let this come to a boil, lower the heat and simmer gently until the potatoes are soft.
- Turn off the heat, and sprinkle the fresh herbs. Cool the mixture and blend until silky smooth. You can do this in batches.

- Once the herbs are fully blended, pour it back into the same pot over low heat. Stir in the almond milk. Gently heat, being careful to not over-simmer. Turn off the heat and let it cool a bit before serving. Eat it warm, not hot.

34. Pumpkin soup

Ingredients

1 tsp olive oil
4–5 garlic cloves, sliced
1 onion, sliced
250 gm pumpkin, chopped
¼ tsp cumin powder
¼ tsp coriander powder
½ tsp turmeric powder
¼ tsp cayenne pepper
3 cups water
Salt to taste
Black pepper crushed for garnish
Coriander leaves for garnish

Method

- In a pressure cooker, on medium heat, add the olive oil and then the garlic. Once the garlic changes colour, add the onions and sauté.
- Then add the pumpkin, cumin, coriander, turmeric powder and cayenne pepper and sauté further.
- Next, add 3 cups of water and salt to taste. Cook for about 3–4 whistles. Once done, grind the same with a hand blender.

- Serve it hot. Garnish it with some freshly ground black pepper and fresh coriander leaves.

35. Leek and romaine lettuce soup

Ingredients

2 tbsp olive oil
½ onion, diced
1–2 fat garlic cloves, roughly chopped
1 cup fresh romaine lettuce leaves, chopped
3 stems leeks, chopped
1 small potato, sliced into ½-inch thick rounds
1 bay leaf (optional, remove before blending)
Salt and pepper to taste
¼ cup fresh dill
½ cup fresh parsley
30 ml almond milk

Method

- Heat oil in a pan and add onions and stir. Now, add the garlic and stir for 1–2 minutes.
- Add the romaine, leeks, potatoes, salt and pepper, and top up with water to cover the vegetables. Let this come to a boil, lower heat and simmer gently until the potatoes are soft.
- Turn the heat off and add the fresh herbs and leave aside to cool.
- Once cooled, blend until silky smooth (about a minute). You can do this in batches. Once the herbs are fully blended, pour it back into the same pot and put it over low heat.

- Stir in the almond milk. Gently heat, being careful to not let it come to a boil. Turn off the heat and let it cool a bit before serving. Eat it warm, not hot.

36. Carrot soup

Ingredients

1 tbsp olive oil
⅓ cup onions, chopped (approx. 60 gm)
3 garlic cloves, chopped
3 medium carrots, chopped into small chunks
Sea salt to taste
2 cups vegetable stock
¼ tsp ground or crushed black pepper
1–2 tbsp of chopped fresh herb such as parsley, coriander, mint, dill leaves, chives or thyme (for garnish)

Method

- Heat olive oil in a pan and add the onions. Sauté on medium heat while stirring often till the onions soften and turn translucent.
- Add the garlic and sauté for about 10–15 seconds or until the raw aroma of garlic goes away.
- Next, add the carrots and season with sea salt to taste. Mix and sauté for a minute.
- Add 1 cup water or vegetable stock. Stir to combine. Cover the pan and simmer on low to medium-low heat, checking intermittently till the carrots are tender and soft.
- Switch off the heat and place the pan on the kitchen countertop to cool. Then transfer the contents of the pan to a blender jar.

- Add ½ cup water or vegetable stock and blend to a smooth and fine purée. Make sure there are no chunks remaining.
- Pour the blended mixture back into the same pan.
- Add ½ cup more water or vegetable stock and mix well. Return the pan to the stovetop again and heat on a low flame. For a thinner consistency, you can add some more water or vegetable stock.
- Once the soup is warm, add black pepper and mix well. Before serving, garnish with any of the listed fresh herbs.

37. Mixed wholesome vegetable soup

Ingredients

1 tbsp rice bran oil

1 medium size onion, chopped

2 garlic cloves, minced

Three days a week, alternating: 1 cup each, shredded carrot, French beans, cabbage

Four days a week, alternating: 1 cup each, shredded carrots, any gourd, 6–7 romaine lettuce leaves

1 cup water

Salt and pepper to taste

5 tbsp boiled quinoa (optional—you can have any of the permitted carbohydrates)

2 tbsp EVOO

Method

- In a pan, add the rice bran oil, onions and garlic. Stir-fry for 5–7 minutes.

- Add the vegetable combination as per days if you are repeating this soup through the week. Stir-fry for a further 5–7 minutes.
- Add 1 cup water and simmer for 7–10 minutes on low flame, keeping the pan covered. Switch off the heat and let the pan sit, still covered, for 30 minutes.
- Next, transfer the contents to a blender and blend till smooth. Add salt and pepper, the boiled quinoa and the EVOO. Serve hot.

Note: In case you are using the combination with romaine lettuce, add the leaves just one minute before you switch off the gas.

38. Chicken noodle soup

Ingredients

4 garlic cloves, sliced and toasted crispy in EVOO (for garnishing)
1 chicken breast with bone
2 cups water
75 gm rice noodles
2 tbsp EVOO
1 cup stir-fried vegetables (see p. 230)
A pinch of ground black pepper
2–3 thyme sprigs
2 garlic cloves, minced
1 tsp chopped fresh parsley or thyme for seasoning

Method

- In a ceramic pan, on low heat, lightly toast the sliced garlic. Switch off the heat and keep the toasted garlic aside.
- Add chicken breast to a pan with 2 cups of water. Simmer on medium heat for 20 minutes, partially covered. This will make the chicken broth (which is different from chicken stock as chicken stock is made primarily from the bones).
- Cook the rice noodles by immersing them in very hot water for three minutes and then draining the water. Run the noodles under cold water, drain and toss with a bit of olive oil.
- In a pan, add the stir-fried vegetables, herbs and spices directly as the stir-fried vegetables are already cooked and we want to sauté till fragrant. Pour the broth over the vegetables, add noodles, cover the pot and turn up the heat for 3–4 minutes. Remove the cooked chicken and dice or shred it and then add it back to the pot. You can make a low-carb version by replacing rice noodles with zucchini.

39. Caesar salad

Ingredients

2 garlic cloves, sliced
Herbs such as chopped coriander, oregano, thyme, rosemary
Salt, pepper and chilli flakes (optional)
2 tbsp EVOO
7–8 pieces romaine lettuce leaves

A spring onion stock or medium-sized regular onion, chopped (optional)
1 grilled chicken breast (optional)
20 gm crumbled vegan almond cheese

Method

- In a pan, toast the sliced garlic and set aside.
- For the dressing, mix the herbs, garlic, salt, pepper and chilli flakes in the EVOO.
- Toss the romaine lettuce, spring onions or onions, grilled chicken (optional) and other ingredients together to make the salad.

40. Healthy potato salad

Ingredients

4 tbsp EVOO
4 tbsp almond butter
2 tbsp almond milk
10–12 pieces romaine lettuce leaves, well washed
1 stalk celery, chopped (optional)
3–4 garlic cloves, minced
2 stalks spring onions, chopped
½ tsp dill
Gluten-free grainy mustard
1 kg boiled potatoes, peeled and kept aside
3 hardboiled eggs (optional, use 75 gm tofu if you don't eat eggs)
½ tsp chilli flakes (optional)
1–2 green chillies (optional)
Salt and pepper to taste

Method

- *For the dressing*: mix the EVOO with the almond butter and almond milk. Add the romaine lettuce, celery, garlic, spring onions, dill and a dash of gluten-free grainy mustard and mix together till smooth and soft. You can also use a whisk.
- Chop the potatoes and hardboiled eggs and arrange them on a serving dish. Add the dressing and mix together with your hands for the eggs and potatoes to be completely coated. Refrigerate and serve cold.

Note: After one year of following my plan, you can also *occasionally* use Greek yoghurt instead of almond butter and almond milk for the dressing.

41. Cucumber salad

Ingredients

2 tbsp fresh chives, finely chopped
2 tbsp EVOO
1½ tsp honey
Salt to taste
Freshly ground pepper to taste
4 medium cucumbers, peeled and cut in cubes
Chia seeds (for garnish, optional)

Method

- Mix all the ingredients (except the cucumbers) and allow the flavours to meld. Then, add cucumbers and serve immediately. Garnish with chia seeds for an extra crunch.

42. Avocado salad

Ingredients

2 tbsp EVOO
Salt and pepper to taste
½ medium onion, finely chopped
2 green chillies, seedless and finely chopped (optional)
1 tsp organic honey
2 tbsp fresh coriander leaves, chopped
½ cup romaine lettuce
1 cup avocado, chopped
1 tbsp toasted almonds, sliced

Method

- Combine EVOO, salt and pepper in a bowl. Let it stand at room temperature for one hour.
- Add onions, green chillies, honey and coriander to the EVOO mix. Mix well.
- Cut the lettuce into thick strips. Arrange lettuce on a platter and top with chopped avocados. Pour the oil mix liberally, sprinkle toasted almonds on the avocados for crunchiness. Serve.

43. Brown rice salad

Ingredients

5 heaped tbsp boiled brown rice
½ onion, chopped
10–12 large romaine lettuce leaves, finely chopped
1 cucumber, finely chopped

15–20 coriander leaves

2 or more green chillies, finely chopped (optional, increase as per taste)

Salt and pepper to taste

½ cup crushed toasted almonds

1 tbsp honey

3 tbsp EVOO

Method

- Mix everything together and leave it in the refrigerator for 30 minutes before serving.

44. Lettuce and papaya salad

Ingredients

1 firm and ripe medium-size papaya, julienned and chopped as per method

3 tbsp EVOO

Salt to taste

A pinch of black pepper, freshly ground

6 cups mixed lettuce and arugula, roughly torn

2 tbsp fresh coriander

2 tbsp almonds, sliced

Method

- Halve, seed and peel the papaya. Cut two-thirds of it into fine julienne strips two inches long. Sprinkle with some of the olive oil. Set aside.

- Roughly chop the remaining papaya and transfer it to a blender along with the remaining olive oil. Blend until smooth and then season with salt and pepper.
- Place the lettuce and coriander in a large bowl. Add the papaya dressing and toss gently. Sprinkle with the julienned papaya and almonds.

45. Egg salad with basil

Ingredients

8–10 basil leaves
2 tbsp EVOO
1 garlic clove, grated
Salt to taste
Pepper, freshly ground
2 hardboiled eggs, quartered
1 carrot, julienned
1 fennel, julienned

Method

- Blend the basil leaves to chutney consistency, then add olive oil, garlic, salt and pepper.
- Arrange eggs, carrots and fennel in a bowl. Drizzle the dressing on top. Serve.

46. Avocado and broccoli warm salad

Ingredients

1 tbsp rice bran oil
1 medium-sized onion, sliced

¼ tsp sea salt

4 garlic cloves, minced

1 head of broccoli, cut into florets (4 cups)

¼ cup water

1 small head of cabbage, sliced into thin ribbons

2 cups well washed rocket leaves

2 tbsp avocado sauce (see next recipe)

2 tbsp toasted sesame seeds, for garnish (optional)

Method

- Heat the rice bran oil in a wok or large skillet over medium heat. Add the onion and salt. Stir-fry for 5 minutes, or until the onion softens.
- Add the garlic and cook for another 2 minutes.
- Then add the broccoli and ¼ cup water. Cover and steam for 3 minutes before adding the cabbage. Steam for 2 more minutes.
- Place 1 cup rocket leaves on a plate. Top with 1 cup broccoli mixture, and drizzle avocado sauce. Sprinkle with sesame seeds.

47. Avocado sauce

Ingredients

1 garlic clove, peeled and sliced

2 soft avocados

1 tbsp cold-pressed olive oil

2 tsp honey

Salt and pepper to taste

½ cup water

Method

- Mince the garlic in a food processor. Add the other ingredients and blend with ½ cup water until smooth. Store in the refrigerator. This sauce can be served with salads.

48. Khichadi

Ingredients

3 tbsp raw quinoa
1 tbsp rice bran oil
1 medium-sized onion, chopped
2 garlic cloves, crushed
Whole spices such as mustard seeds, cumin seeds, cardamom and cloves, as per taste
3 cups different permitted vegetables
1 tbsp raw white rice
Salt and pepper to taste

Method

- In a pressure cooker, add the rice bran oil, onion, garlic and whole spices as per taste. Add the quinoa, vegetables, rice, salt and pepper with some water. Pressure cook for 1 whistle, then reduce the heat. Cook for another 20 minutes then switch off the heat. Don't touch the cooker or whistle for 45 minutes. This preserves the water-soluble vitamins.
- Open the cooker without taking off the whistle, mix well and serve hot. The ratio of vegetables to rice after cooking should be 50:50. In case you want your khichadi even softer,

you can cook for an extra 10 minutes in the pressure cooker. You can also blend it for easier swallowing and absorption.

49. Gourd curry

Ingredients

1 tsp rice bran oil
1 medium-sized onion, chopped
2 garlic cloves, grated
1 tsp mustard seeds or 1 tsp cumin seeds
5 curry leaves (optional)
1 cup each, any three permitted vegetables
½ cup gourd*
Salt to taste
½ tsp organic turmeric powder
A pinch of black pepper
A few coriander leaves

*Choose one of any one of these gourds as per availability: bottle gourd (*lauki*), ridge gourd (*tori*), pointed gourd (*parmal*), round gourd (*tinda*) or pumpkin.

Method

- In a pressure cooker, add the rice bran oil and the onion and stir-fry for 5 minutes.
- Add mustard or cumin seeds and optional curry leaves and stir-fry for another 5 minutes on high heat.
- Add grated garlic, stir-fry for another 2 minutes.
- Add the vegetables, turmeric, black pepper and salt to taste. Don't add water. Close the pressure cooker and cook for 2 whistles before switching off the heat. Don't touch or open

the pressure cooker for 45 minutes. This preserves the water-soluble vitamins. Open and serve hot.

50. Stir-fried vegetables

Ingredients

1 cup carrots, shredded
1 cup French beans, thinly sliced
½ cup fresh or frozen peas
1 tbsp EVOO
3 garlic cloves, crushed
1 medium-sized onion, finely chopped
2 sliced green chillies (optional)
Salt and pepper to taste
A pinch of organic turmeric powder

Method

- Finely slice the above or other permitted vegetables.
- Add 1 tablespoon EVOO to a pan. Add three crushed garlic cloves and stir-fry.
- Add onions and sliced green chilies, stir-fry for another minute before adding the vegetables. Cook for 5 minutes then add salt, a pinch of black pepper, a pinch of turmeric powder. Reduce the flame, cover with lid and switch off the heat.
- Don't cook for more than 5 minutes as the vegetables need to be crunchy. If you have a gut issue, you can cook them longer; otherwise vegetables that are slightly crunchy have a higher nutritive value. Allow to cool while still covered.

The water-soluble vitamins in the vegetables will get destroyed if the lid is open.

51. Coriander curry

Ingredients

2 tbsp rice bran oil
3 onions, peeled and chopped
10 curry leaves
5 garlic cloves, peeled and chopped
30–40 coriander leaves, chopped
1 tsp cumin seeds
2 green chillies, cut lengthwise (optional)
½ tsp turmeric powder
Salt and pepper to taste

Method

- In a ceramic pan, on medium heat, add a tablespoon of rice bran oil. Then add the onions, curry leaves and garlic and stir-fry till golden-brown.
- Add the coriander leaves and stir-fry for 5 minutes before switching off the heat. Let it cool and then add to a blender with a little water. Blend well and leave aside.
- In a small pan, heat a tablespoon of rice bran oil, then add the cumin seeds, green chillies and turmeric powder. Stir-fry for 5 minutes. Add salt and pepper and mix with the coriander paste.
- Add this to a pressure cooker and dilute with water to make it into the base for a vegetable curry. You can add permitted

vegetables. Close the pressure cooker and give it 2 whistles and turn off the heat. You can also use this curry base in a wide pan and add permitted vegetables of choice and simmer till crunchy but soft, for 5–7 minutes with the pan lid covered.

52. Tofu bhurji

Ingredients

200 gm firm tofu
1 tbsp rice bran oil
1 medium-sized onion, finely chopped
1 tsp cumin seeds
2 green chillies, finely chopped (optional)
10–12 coriander leaves, finely chopped
½ tsp turmeric powder
A pinch of black pepper
Sea salt to taste

Method

- Crumble the tofu with your hands. Keep aside and cover.
- In a pan, on medium heat, add the rice bran oil, onions and cumin seeds and sauté for 2 minutes.
- Then add the green chillies, coriander leaves, turmeric powder, black pepper and salt. Sauté for another minute before adding the crumbled tofu. Stir the mixture for 2–3 minutes till everything is mixed together and the tofu is properly coated with the turmeric. Serve hot.

53. Rice-stuffed cabbage rolls

Ingredients

    2 cups cooked brown and white rice mixed
    Rice bran oil to pan-fry
    ½ cup onion, finely chopped
    1 garlic clove, minced
    1 cup broccoli or cauliflower
    1 cup carrot, finely chopped
    1 cup French beans, finely chopped
    Salt to taste
    ¼ tsp turmeric powder
    1 pinch of black pepper
    ¼ tsp cumin seeds
    3–4 big leaves of cabbage

Method

- Cook brown and white rice in an equal proportion. Keep aside.
- In a pan, on medium heat, add a little oil and then the onion, garlic, broccoli, carrots and French beans and sauté. Add salt, turmeric and black pepper. Keep aside.
- In another pan, heat a small amount of rice bran oil and add the cumin seeds. Switch off the heat once the cumin seeds start crackling. Add this seasoning to the boiled brown and white rice mixture. Keep aside.
- Blanch the cabbage leaves by putting them in boiling water for a minute and then immersing them in cold water. This helps maintain the colour of the leaves. Knife the thick white centre from the cabbage leaves, in a V-shaped cut.

- Spread a layer of rice mixture over a cabbage leaf and add an equal amount of sautéed vegetables over it. Pull together the cut edges of the cabbage leaf, fold over filling, tuck in the sides and roll it. Repeat for all the cabbage leaves.

Note: In case you need to increase your protein intake, add crumbled tofu or tofu bhurji instead of the rice.

54. Rice wrap

Ingredients

2 tbsp rice flour
1 tbsp psyllium husk
1 potato, half-boiled
1 onion, chopped
Salt to taste

Method

- Knead rice flour, psyllium husk, boiled potato and chopped onion together. Add salt to taste.
- Shape into a pancake with your hands. Don't use a rolling pin or it will break. You can use white rice flour to dust it while rolling.
- Heat a flat pan and dry roast the pancake on each side until golden-brown.
- Serve with EVOO and stir-fried vegetables.

55. Vegetable curry

Ingredients

1 tbsp rice bran oil
1 medium-sized onion, chopped

2 garlic cloves, grated
1 tsp mustard seeds or 1 tsp cumin seeds
5 curry leaves (optional)
1 cup each, any three permitted vegetables
½ tsp turmeric
A pinch of black pepper
Salt to taste
12–15 coriander leaves

Method

- In a pressure cooker, add the rice bran oil, onion and garlic and stir-fry for 5 minutes.
- Add mustard or cumin seeds and optional curry leaves and stir-fry for another 5 minutes on high heat. Add the vegetables, turmeric, black pepper and salt to taste. Don't add water. Close the pressure cooker and cook it for 2 whistles before switching off the heat. Don't open the pressure cooker for 45 minutes. This preserves the water-soluble vitamins. Open and serve hot.

56. Quinoa flour roti

Ingredients

2 tbsp quinoa flour
1 tbsp psyllium husk
1 potato, half-boiled
1 onion, chopped (optional)
8–10 washed coriander leaves
A pinch of ajwain
Salt to taste

Method

- Knead all ingredients listed together. Make into a flat shape with your hands. Don't use a rolling pin or it will break. You can use rice flour to dust it while rolling.
- Cook on a flat pan, on medium heat, until golden-brown on both sides. Serve with EVOO.

57. Rice flour roti

Ingredients

2 tbsp rice flour
1 tbsp psyllium husk
1 potato, half-boiled
1 onion, chopped (optional)
1 tbsp grated bottle gourd
Salt to taste

Method

- Knead all the ingredients together. Make into a flat shape with your hands. Don't use a rolling pin or it will break. You can use rice flour to dust it while rolling.
- Cook on a flat pan, on medium heat, until golden-brown on both sides. Serve with EVOO.

58. Brown rice flour roti

Ingredients

2 tbsp brown rice flour
1 tbsp psyllium husk
1 potato, half-boiled

1 onion, chopped
8–10 coriander leaves
A pinch of ajwain
Salt to taste

Method

- Knead all the ingredients together. Make into a flat shape with your hands. Don't use a rolling pin or it will break. You can use rice flour to dust it while rolling.
- Cook on a flat pan, on medium heat, until golden-brown on both sides. Serve with EVOO.

59. Amaranth flour roti

Ingredients

2 tbsp amaranth flour
1 tbsp psyllium husk
1 potato, half-boiled
1 onion, chopped
12–15 washed coriander leaves
A pinch of roasted jeera
Salt to taste

Method

- Knead all ingredients together. Make into a flat shape with your hands. Don't use a rolling pin or it will break. You can use rice flour to dust it while rolling.
- Cook on a flat pan, on medium heat, until golden-brown on both sides. Serve with EVOO.

60. Almond flour paratha

Ingredients

    2 tbsp almond flour
    1 tbsp psyllium husk
    1 potato, half-boiled
    1 onion, chopped
    1 stalk well washed coriander leaves
    A pinch of ajwain
    Salt to taste

Method

- Knead all ingredients together. Make into a flat shape with your hands. Don't use a rolling pin or it will break. You can use rice flour to dust it while rolling.
- Cook on a flat pan, on medium heat, until golden-brown on both sides. Serve with EVOO.

61. Tofu cutlet

Ingredients

    2 tbsp peas
    1 small zucchini, grated
    30 gm pressure cooker boiled white rice
    ½ medium-sized potato, boiled and mashed
    100 gm tofu, crumbled
    1 spring onion, finely chopped
    5–6 basil leaves, crushed

½ tsp garlic paste
¼ tsp red chilli flakes (optional)
1 tsp white sesame seeds
Salt and pepper to taste
¼ tsp turmeric powder
2 tbsp rice bran oil

Method

- Parboil the peas and zucchini by running them through hot water, draining and covering them for 10 minutes.
- Add all the ingredients listed and mash together.
- Add salt, pepper and turmeric powder and shallow fry in rice bran oil on high heat till crisp on each side.

62. Veg cutlet

Ingredients

1 spring onion, finely chopped
½ cup cabbage, shredded
1 tbsp peas
30 gm quinoa, pressure-cooked
2 medium-sized potatoes, boiled and mashed
5–6 mint leaves, finely chopped
½ tsp garlic paste
¼ tsp red chilli powder (optional)
Salt and pepper to taste
¼ tsp turmeric powder
2 tbsp rice bran oil

Method

- Parboil the raw vegetables by running them through hot water, draining and covering them for 10 minutes. Mash together with the quinoa and potatoes.
- Add garlic paste, mint leaves, chilli powder, salt, pepper and turmeric powder and shallow fry in rice bran oil on high heat till crisp on each side.

63. Sweet potato chaat

Ingredients

100 gm sweet potato
½ medium-sized onion, chopped
1–2 green chillies (optional)
1 tbsp coriander chutney (see p. 204)
10 mint leaves, finely chopped
A pinch of black pepper
1 tbsp EVOO
Salt to taste

Method

- Boil the sweet potato. Allow it to cool. Peel and chop it and then mix well with all the other ingredients listed. You can also add romaine and cucumber and have it as a side portion or salad.

64. Thai green curry

Ingredients

For the curry paste
5 curry leaves
3 green chillies, chopped
¼ cup coriander leaves, chopped
3 basil leaves
1 tbsp coriander seeds, whole roasted
1 tsp cumin seeds, roasted
1 tsp black peppercorns
1 onion, roughly chopped
¼ cup spring onion, roughly chopped
3 garlic cloves
Salt to taste

For the curry
1 tsp rice bran oil
1 cup broccoli florets
1 carrot, sliced
½ cup French beans, cut into long slices
½ green zucchini, quartered or thickly sliced
3 tbsp curry paste (made with ingredients above)
1 cup vegetable stock
1 tbsp brown sugar
400 ml unsweetened almond milk

Salt to taste
1 basil leaf

Method

- Blend all the ingredients for the curry paste with a little bit of water into a smooth paste. Store it in a glass jar.
- On the stove, place a wok and heat oil. Add the broccoli, carrots, French beans, zucchini and salt. Stir-fry on high heat until slightly tender. Remove from the wok and keep aside.
- Add the oil and curry paste into the hot wok and sauté for a few seconds. Add the vegetable stock or water and stir, then add the brown sugar and finally the almond milk. Stir to combine all the ingredients. Once combined, add some salt and allow the mixture to thicken a little and come to a boil.
- When it is boiling, add in the basil leaf and the stir-fried vegetables kept aside earlier. Mix well.
- Serve with a bowl of white or jasmine rice (see next recipe).

65. Jasmine rice

Ingredients

1 cup short-grain rice (like Japanese rice)
1 teabag of jasmine tea

Method

- It's very important to not use water in a quantity double that of the rice as we normally use for cooking white rice. Use 1.5x the amount to make it sticky like in restaurants. Wash the rice 3–4 times, not more. Don't soak. Add 1½ cups of water to the rice. Cook in semi-covered pan on medium to low heat.

- After 7–8 minutes, add the jasmine tea bag to the rice.
- After another 2–3 minutes, when the rice isn't yet completely cooked, switch off the heat and cover completely. Only open after 30 minutes. This is a very important step to get the sticky fragrant restaurant-like jasmine rice. Serve with Thai green curry (see previous recipe).

66. Singapore noodles

Ingredients

2.5 l water

100 gm thin rice noodles

1 tbsp Chinese sesame oil* (optional)

Half cup each red cabbage, carrots, French beans, finely sliced

1 onion, finely sliced

6–7 garlic cloves, peeled and ground coarsely

Salt to taste

Black pepper to taste

Chilli flakes for sprinkling to taste (optional)

*The Chinese sesame oil adds a nutty flavour to the dish. If you prefer a different flavour, replace the oil with your choice of herb from rosemary, oregano or thyme.

Method

- Bring 2.5 litres of water to a boil, add the rice noodles, stir for 5 minutes and then switch off the heat. Rice noodles take very little time to cook so make sure that you are monitoring it closely. Drain the water using a sieve. Wash the rice noodles under cold running water then cover and put aside.

- In a ceramic pan, add the sesame oil (or herbs), vegetables and garlic. Stir-fry for 5 minutes while adding salt to taste. Switch off the heat, cover tightly and let it sit for 10 minutes. This helps better absorption of water-soluble vitamins.
- After 10 minutes, put it back on the heat. Remove the lid and add the black pepper and chilli flakes. Stir in the cooked rice noodles. Mix them well together with two wooden ladles so that the rice noodles are handled delicately and don't break.

67. Pesto sauce

Ingredients

10–12 basil leaves
30 coriander leaves
3 medium-sized garlic cloves, peeled
30 pine nuts
4 tbsp EVOO
Salt, pepper, herbs to taste

Method

- Wash the basil and coriander leaves very thoroughly, then soak for five minutes in water with a spoon of salt dissolved in it. Drain.
- Add all the ingredients listed with some water in a blender and blend to a chutney consistency.
- Add salt, pepper and herbs and mix well with a spoon. This pesto sauce is okay to refrigerate for up to three days.

68. Pizza base

Ingredients

2 large potatoes
⅓ cup warm water
1 tbsp honey
7–8 grams dry yeast
½ cup tapioca starch
1 cup white rice flour
⅓ tsp salt
1 large egg white
1 tbsp EVOO

Method

- Boil the potatoes in a pressure cooker and allow to cool. Peel and mash them. Set aside.
- Mix the warm water, honey and yeast in a measuring cup or small bowl. Let it sit for 3–5 minutes until a small layer of foam develops at the top. If this doesn't happen, discard and try again with fresher yeast.
- Mix potatoes, tapioca starch, rice flour and salt in a bowl. Knead with your hands or in a food processor on medium speed until the mixture is combined and forms a fine, crumbly dough.
- Add the egg white and EVOO, slowly drizzle in the yeast mixture and mix. Cover with a cloth and set aside for 1½ hours. The dough will rise by half.
- Now your pizza base is ready to be put into the oven with permitted toppings of your choice.

- Heat oven for 10 minutes at 180°C.
- Bake at 180°C for 10 minutes or less—keep checking to get the crispness you want.

69. Cauliflower pizza base

Ingredients

2 cups water
2 cups cauliflower, grated
1 egg, beaten
1 tsp dried oregano
1 tsp dried parsley
1 garlic clove, minced
½ cup grated vegan cheese (see p. 208)
2 tbsp olive oil
Sea salt
Freshly ground black pepper

Method

- Preheat the oven to 200°C.
- Fill a pan with 2 cups of water and bring it to a light boil over medium heat.
- Add the grated cauliflower and let it cook for 4–5 minutes. Drain the water from the saucepan. Drain cauliflower through a cheesecloth, squeezing it tightly. Remove as much water as possible. Allow cauliflower to cool.
- Meanwhile, in a bowl, beat an egg and mix in dried herbs and garlic. Add olive oil as you mix everything. Add salt and pepper.

- On a baking tray lined with parchment paper, spread the dough and shape it into a round shape. Sprinkle vegan cheese on it.
- Bake in the oven for 15–20 minutes. Switch off the oven and leave the pizza base inside for 5 more minutes then take it out. Enjoy!

70. Mashed potatoes

Ingredients

3 medium-sized boiled potatoes, peeled and mashed
Salt and pepper to taste
EVOO
Seasonings such as dill, oregano, thyme, rosemary or cracked pepper to taste

Method

- Mash everything together. Add 2 tablespoons of the EVOO per serving and garnish with seasonings of your choice.

71. Broccoli tofu stir-fry

Ingredients

1 cup broccoli, chopped
200 gm firm tofu
Salt and pepper to taste
1 tbsp EVOO
1 tbsp rice bran oil
1 cup spring onions, sliced
1 tbsp soy sauce

1 tsp sesame oil
1 tbsp toasted sesame seeds
1 tbsp honey (optional)

Method

- Boil some water and add the broccoli in it for just two minutes. Drain and run the broccoli under cold water to keep it crispy.
- Cut the tofu into medium-sized squares.
- Put a wok on high heat and add EVOO. Toss in the tofu and stir-fry till it becomes golden and crispy. Keep aside.
- In the same wok, add rice bran oil and lightly stir-fry the green onions. Don't brown them.
- Add the broccoli, soy sauce, sesame oil, salt and pepper. Stir-fry for another minute before returning the crispy tofu to the wok. After a minute, switch off the heat and sprinkle the toasted sesame seeds on the dish.
- You can add honey if you want a sweeter taste. Serve hot with rice porridge or steamed jasmine rice.

72. Soy nuggets curry

Ingredients

4 tbsp dehydrated soy granules or nuggets
1 tbsp rice bran oil
1 medium-sized onion, chopped
2 garlic cloves, grated
1 tsp mustard seeds or cumin seeds
½ tsp turmeric powder
A pinch of black pepper

Salt to taste
1 tbsp peas
10–12 coriander leaves
5 curry leaves (optional)

Method

- Soak the soy nuggets for 1 hour.
- In a pan, add a teaspoon of rice bran oil and roast the onion and garlic till brown. Set aside and allow it to cool. Once cool, blend it into a paste.
- Temper mustard or cumin seeds with curry leaves in a teaspoon of rice bran oil and stir-fry for 5 minutes on high heat.
- Drain the soy nuggets, squeeze out any excess water.
- In a pan, add 1 cup water with the turmeric, black pepper, and the onion and garlic paste. Mix well, then add salt, soy nuggets and peas.
- Simmer for 10–15 minutes. Add the tempering of mustard or cumin seeds with curry leaves. Garnish with coriander leaves and serve.

73. Roasted beans

This recipe can be used for French beans, flat beans, asparagus or green beans of any kind.

Ingredients

2 tbsp EVOO
3 cloves garlic, minced
1 onion, chopped

250 gm French beans or any green beans
A pinch of turmeric
Salt and pepper to taste

Method

- Stir-fry the onion and garlic in EVOO on low heat and keep aside.
- French beans have a tough, woody end that should be removed before roasting. Bend the sides of the French beans and the beans will naturally snap in the right place. Hold the entire bunch of French beans in one hand (this works very well if you use a rubber band to bunch them together) and trim off the bottoms by about 1.5 inches.
- Wash and dry the French beans. You can do this either before or after trimming it; just be sure to dry it completely. Add a light coating of EVOO on the beans. Keep the seasonings simple with a dash of turmeric, salt and pepper. If you want to flavour with some rosemary, thyme, oregano and sprinkled chilli flakes, that is also fine.
- Spread the beans in a single layer in an oven dish, so that they can be evenly roasted in the oven. Roast at 200°C. Make sure that you check on them every 5 minutes as beans don't take very long to cook. If you don't have an oven, you can cover the pan with a dome-shaped lid and put it on medium heat. Sauté for 3–4 minutes till they become golden-brown and crispy.
- Once done, season with the garlic and onions by sprinkling it on top before serving. This particular dish can be combined with various kinds of cuisines or be served as a snack with mulled wine.

74. Chicken meatballs

Ingredients

2 eggs
2 tbsp EVOO
Salt, pepper, herbs to taste
½ kg chicken, minced
10–12 coriander leaves, finely chopped
Herbs such as dill, rosemary, oregano, thyme (optional)
Gluten free breadcrumbs (optional)

Method

- Preheat the oven to 200°C.
- Beat the eggs. Add EVOO, salt, pepper, minced chicken and coriander leaves. You can add other herbs or chilli flakes for flavour (optional). Gently mix together, and shape into balls. Roll in breadcrumbs (optional).
- Line an oven tray with aluminium foil and arrange the meatballs on it. Brush with EVOO and roast for 20 minutes. Ensure it doesn't burn. You can poke the meatballs with a fork to check if they're done inside.
- Serve with spaghetti, mashed potatoes or with a side of vegetables and salad.

75. Fish kebabs

Ingredients

½ kg salmon fillet
½ cup water

8 garlic cloves
1 onion
½ tsp red chilli powder (optional)
A pinch of turmeric powder
Salt and pepper
1 slice gluten-free bread

For sautéing
1 tbsp rice bran oil
½ tbsp garlic paste
1 onion, finely chopped
2 green chillies, finely chopped (optional)
2 tbsp fresh coriander leaves

Method

- In a pan, put the fish fillet with ½ cup water, garlic, onion, red chilli powder, turmeric powder, salt and pepper and steam on low heat for 5 minutes. Switch off the heat and keep aside.
- Mince the above in a grinder.
- Heat oil in a pan and sauté the garlic paste, onion and green chillies on high heat for 2–3 minutes. Add coriander leaves and the fish mince.
- Roll into kebabs. Roll in rice flour if unable to shape them.
- Shallow fry on a pan or air-fry at 180°C on level 6—the fish is already cooked so all you need to do is to make it crisp. Keep the heat high. You can also put the kebabs for 5 minutes in an oven preheated to 200°C. You can also combine this with brown sauce (see next recipe), steamed rice and mashed potatoes.

76. Brown sauce

Ingredients

   1 chicken breast or 150 gm fish or 150 gm tofu
   1 tbsp rice bran oil
   1 tbsp almond butter
   8–10 button mushrooms (for those with thyroid issues, you can use 7–8 caramelized onions)
   2 cloves garlic, minced
   200 ml chicken or vegetable broth
   1 tsp rice flour for thickening, or as required
   200 ml chicken or vegetable broth

Method

- Pan-fry chicken breast, fish or tofu and keep aside.
- *For fish and tofu:* Add 1 tablespoon rice bran oil and pan-fry the same on high heat for 3 minutes each side till crisp and brown, and keep aside.
- *For chicken breast:* Pan-fry the chicken on high heat till it turns crisp and brown and then reduce the heat, add a little bit of water to cover the breast, cover the pan with the lid and simmer till the chicken becomes tender. Keep checking on it with a fork.
- *For the sauce:* Add almond butter to a pan with mushrooms or onions and cook for 3 minutes or until golden. Add more butter and garlic. Cook for a minute and then turn the heat down.
- Add 1 teaspoon of rice flour and mix for a minute.

- Mix chicken or vegetable broth gradually into this. Stir constantly to avoid lumps. Use a whisk if needed. Cook for about 2 minutes or until it thickens. It will thicken more as it cools. Add salt and pepper. If you want the sauce to be smooth, let it cool and then blend till smooth while adding a bit of stock.
- As the sauce gets ready, add chicken, fish or tofu on the pan and coat in the sauce, and simmer for 7–8 minutes. Add water if you want a thinner consistency. Switch off the heat and allow the protein to absorb the sauce for 7–8 minutes.
- This is best served with mashed potato and vegetables/salads.

77. Chinese fried rice

For crispy Chinese fried rice, use cold, leftover cooked rice. You can make veg or non-veg versions as per your preference.

Ingredients

200 gm minced chicken or crumbled tofu or sliced salmon

½ cup carrot, shredded

4 tbsp frozen or fresh peas

½ cup cabbage, shredded

2 tbsp EVOO

½ cup spring onions, sliced

10–12 garlic cloves, sliced

Boiled rice as per your hunger/serving size. Ideally it should be 25 per cent of the entire meal on your plate.

Salt and pepper to taste

2 eggs

1 tsp sesame oil

Method

- Season the meat, fish or tofu with salt and pepper in a bowl.
- Boil water in a pan. Add all the vegetables. Boil for 3–4 minutes on high heat and then strain and run the vegetables under cold water. Keep aside.
- In a pan, add 1 tablespoon of EVOO, spring onions and garlic and stir-fry.
- Add the rice, stirring to break up clumps. Mix well with the spring onions and garlic and push to the side of the pan.
- Add 1 more tablespoon of EVOO, break in 2 eggs and stir till scrambled. Then add the sesame oil. Serve hot.

78. Grilled coriander fish

Ingredients

30–40 coriander leaves as per how intense you want the coriander flavour

10–12 garlic cloves

2 tbsp rice bran oil

5–6 medium pieces of any oily fish like salmon, rawas (Indian salmon), mackerel, tuna (not canned), anchovies, herring, trout, sardines—as per availability or taste.

½ tsp black pepper

Salt to taste

Method

- Crush the coriander leaves, garlic and oil to a coarse mixture. Alternatively, make a paste by adding a little water.
- In a bowl, add the fish pieces and the coriander mixture and sprinkle black pepper and salt to taste.

- Brush a grill pan with a little oil and switch on the heat. Add the fish-coriander mix and grill each side for 5–7 minutes.
- You can also use an oven. Preheat to 190°C and grill for 10 minutes on each side.

79. Veg quinoa pulao

Ingredients

4 tbsp raw quinoa
2 tbsp white rice
1 tbsp rice bran oil
2 onions
4 whole garlic cloves
1 tsp cumin seeds
1 tsp fenugreek seeds
½ tsp turmeric
A pinch of black pepper or as per intensity of the flavour you desire
2 cloves
1 bay leaf
2 cardamoms
1 cup each of 4 seasonal vegetables
2 cups water
Salt to taste

Method

- Wash the quinoa and rice under cold running water till water runs clear. Put in a large bowl and add water. Soak for 15–20 minutes.

- In a pressure cooker, add the oil, onions and whole garlic cloves and sauté for 1–2 minutes on high heat. Then add all the spices. After they have tempered for a couple of minutes, add the vegetables, mix well and cook for 2 minutes.
- Now add the drained quinoa and mix. Cook for 2 minutes. Add 2 cups water and salt.
- Put the lid on the pressure cooker and cook on medium-high heat for 2 whistles, then reduce the heat. Cook for 10 minutes and then switch off the heat. Allow the pressure cooker to cool for 45 minutes and then open the lid.
- Fluff up the pulao using a fork.

80. Chicken biryani

Ingredients

4 tbsp raw Basmati rice

1 tbsp rice bran oil

2 medium-sized onions, sliced

4 garlic cloves

1 tsp cumin seeds

1 tsp fenugreek seeds

½ tsp turmeric

Black pepper to taste

2 cloves

1 bay leaf

2 cardamoms

2 chicken breasts (1 per person)

1 cup each of any 3 permitted vegetables (cauliflower, broccoli, cabbage, carrot or celery)

Method

- Wash the rice under cold running water till the water runs clear. In a large bowl, add more water and soak the rice for 15–20 minutes.
- In a pressure cooker, add the oil and onions, let them sweat for 45–60 seconds on high heat, then add garlic and sauté till golden-brown. Then add the spices. After they have tempered for a couple of minutes, add the chicken breast and sear on high flame for 5 minutes or till golden-brown.
- Add the vegetables, mix well and cook for 2 minutes. Now add the drained rice and mix. Cook for 2 minutes. Add a cup of water and salt. Put the lid on the pressure cooker and cook on medium-high heat for 2 whistles, then reduce the heat. Cook for 5 minutes and then switch off the heat. Allow the pressure cooker to cool for 45 minutes and then open the lid. Fluff up the rice using a fork.

81. Veg nourishing pot

Ingredients

1 tbsp rice bran
3 garlic cloves, minced (about 1 tbsp)
1 small onion (about ½ cup sliced)
¼ cup water
10 tbsp stir-fried vegetables (see p. 230)
1–2 green chillies sliced (optional)
A handful each of the following: coriander, basil and mint leaves
2 tbsp EVOO

Method

- Heat the rice bran oil in a deep pan over medium-high heat. Add the garlic and onion and sauté until golden-brown, or about 2 minutes.
- Add the water, sliced green chillies and stir-fried vegetables. Reduce heat and simmer for 5 minutes.
- Add the coriander, basil and mint leaves. Mix them in and switch off the heat.
- Serve on 6–7 tablespoons of jasmine rice and add the EVOO.

82. Fish nourishing pot

Ingredients

1 tbsp rice bran oil

1 small onion (about ½ cup sliced)

3 garlic cloves, minced (about 1 tbsp)

1 small onion (about ½ cup sliced)

200 gm fillet of cod, sole or salmon

¼ cup water

7 tbsp stir-fried vegetables (see p. 230)

A handful of coriander leaves

8–10 romaine lettuce leaves

1 tsp chilli (optional)

2 tbsp EVOO

A handful each of the following: basil and mint leaves

Method

- Heat the rice bran oil in a deep pan over medium-high heat. Add the garlic and onion. Stir until golden-brown, or about 2 minutes.
- Add the fish pieces and cook until they turn opaque, flipping them once.
- Add the water and the stir-fried vegetables. Reduce heat and simmer for 5 minutes.
- Add the coriander leaves and romaine lettuce. Mix them in and switch off the heat.
- Serve on top of 6–7 tablespoons of jasmine rice or rice noodles and add the EVOO, basil and mint leaves.

83. Tofu nourishing pot

Ingredients

4–5 romaine lettuce leaves
7 tbsp stir-fried vegetables (see p. 230)
1 tbsp rice bran oil
3 garlic cloves, minced (about 1 tbsp)
1 small onion (about ½ cup sliced)
¼ cup water
Broccoli tofu stir-fry (see p. 247; 1 cup serves 1 person.)
2 tbsp EVOO
1 tsp chilli (optional)
A handful each of the following: basil, coriander and mint leaves

Method

- Heat oil in a deep pan over medium heat. Add the garlic and onion. Stir for 2 minutes.
- Add the water and the broccoli tofu stir-fry. Reduce heat and stir for about 5 minutes.
- Add the coriander leaves and romaine lettuce. Mix them in and switch off the heat.
- Serve with jasmine rice or Singapore noodles and add the EVOO, basil and mint leaves.

84. Almond milk rice meal

Ingredients

1 big onion, thinly sliced
3 cups mixed vegetables (beans, cauliflower, cabbage, carrot, cut in cubes)
½ cup brown rice
½ cup white rice
½ tsp turmeric powder
5 peppercorns
8 mint leaves
1 tbsp coriander leaves
¾ cup almond milk
¾ cup water
Salt to taste

For tempering
1 tbsp rice bran oil

1 piece cinnamon
4 cloves
2 cardamoms
4 bay leaves

For grinding
1 tsp fennel seeds
4 garlic cloves
1 green chilli
1 tsp mace
2 tbsp water

Method

- Heat 1 tablespoon oil in a pressure cooker and then add all the ingredients under 'tempering'. Add the onion and sauté it till the raw smell goes away.
- Add all the ingredients under 'grinding', all the vegetables, turmeric, peppercorns, mint and coriander leaves. Mix well for 1 minute, then add the rice, almond milk, ¾ cup water and salt. Cook for 20 minutes over low heat. Switch off the heat and allow to cool for 30 minutes. Open and fluff the rice.
- This can be a heavy lunch for those who can't add tofu, eggs, chicken or fish to their meals. The almond milk provides richness and protein.

85. Chicken nourishing pot

Ingredients

1 tbsp rice bran oil

3 garlic cloves, minced (about 1 tbsp)

1 small onion (about ½ cup sliced)

200 gm boneless chicken breast, cut into bite-sized pieces

7 tbsp stir-fried vegetables (see p. 230)

8–10 romaine lettuce leaves

¼ cup water

2–3 green chillies, chopped

2 tbsp EVOO

A handful each of basil and parsley leaves

Method

- Heat oil in a deep pan over medium heat. Add the garlic and onion. Stir for 2 minutes, then add the chicken pieces. Cook until they become opaque, flipping them once.
- Add the green chillies, stir gently and then add the water and the stir-fried vegetables. Reduce the heat, and simmer for 5 minutes.
- Add the basil and parsley leaves and romaine lettuce. Mix them in and switch off the heat.
- Serve with jasmine rice and EVOO, basil and mint leaves.

86. Garlic chilli

Ingredients

100 gm dried chillies

10 garlic cloves, minced

15 ml apple juice

Salt and pepper to taste

Method

- Blend all the ingredients together until smooth. Add water if it's too sticky.
- Transfer this mixture to a pan. Simmer for 10 minutes on medium heat to blend the flavours. Adjust salt and pepper as per taste. Cool and transfer to a glass jar. Store in the fridge.

87. Roasted chivda

Ingredients

1 tbsp rice bran oil
1 tbsp mustard seeds
15 curry leaves
6 small whole garlic cloves
½ tsp turmeric powder
A pinch of black pepper
250 gm thin poha
Salt to taste

Method

- Heat a pan, add the rice bran oil, mustard seeds and curry leaves, followed by the garlic. Cook till golden-brown. Add the turmeric and black pepper and stir.
- Next, add the poha and switch to high heat for 5 minutes. Roast well, switch off the heat but keep the pan on the stove for another 5 minutes while stirring a couple of times even with the flame off. Allow the mixture to cool then add salt. Don't add salt before as this can make the poha soggy. Store in a glass jar.

88. Roasted makhanas

Ingredients

1 tbsp rice bran oil
1 tbsp mustard seeds
15 curry leaves
½ tsp turmeric powder
A pinch of black pepper
250 gm foxnuts
Salt to taste

Method

- Heat a pan, add the rice bran oil, mustard seeds and curry leaves. Cook till mustard seeds start popping. Add the turmeric and black pepper and stir.
- Next, add the foxnuts and roast on low heat until golden-brown for 7–9 minutes. Switch off the heat but keep the pan on the stove for another 8–10 minutes. Allow the mixture to cool then add salt. Don't add salt before as this can make the foxnuts soggy. Store in a glass jar.

89. Murmura bhel

Ingredients

1 tbsp mustard seeds
15 curry leaves
½ tsp turmeric powder
A pinch of black pepper
250 gm puffed rice
Salt to taste

Method

- In a pan, on a medium heat, add mustard seeds and curry leaves and stir-fry for 2 minutes or till mustard seeds start popping. Add the turmeric and black pepper and stir.
- Next, add the puffed rice and keep roasting for another 5 minutes or till the rice is golden-brown. Allow the mixture to cool then add salt. Don't add salt before as this can make the puffed rice soggy. Store in a glass jar.

90. Zucchini fries

Ingredients

2 zucchinis
2 eggs
½ cup grated vegan cheese (see p. 208)
¼ cup rice flour
½ tsp oregano
½ tsp garlic powder
½ tsp chilli flakes
Sea salt
Freshly ground black pepper

Method

- Preheat oven to 220°C.
- Slice the zucchinis into 16–18 sticks, each about 4 inches long. Keep aside.
- Beat the eggs in a bowl for about 30 seconds and keep aside.
- In a separate bowl, mix vegan cheese, rice flour, oregano, sea salt, garlic and chilli flakes.

- Coat zucchini slices with the beaten eggs, then dust with the cheese and rice flour mixture.
- Finally, place the coated zucchini sticks on a baking sheet. Bake in the oven for 18–20 minutes, turning them halfway through.

91. Hara amaranth kebabs

Amaranth is high in protein and ideal for those who want to add protein to their diet while avoiding lentils, pulses, milk and milk products.

Ingredients

100 gm amaranth seeds

200 ml water

2 onions, chopped

30–40 fenugreek leaves, chopped (you can increase the quantity of fenugreek leaves if you want a higher intensity of flavour.)

20–30 coriander leaves, chopped

2 green chillies (optional)

3 tbsp of bajra (millet flour), roasted

Salt to taste

Method

- In a pressure cooker, add 200 ml water and the amaranth seeds and give it 1 whistle. Reduce the heat, cook for 20 minutes on low flame and switch off the stove. Allow it to cool.
- Remove the amaranth seeds from the cooker and add to the onions and fenugreek and coriander leaves. Add salt and

green chillies (optional), then knead in 2–3 tablespoons of roasted millet flour to bind.
- Shape into kebabs and pan-fry.

92. Gluten-free crackers

Ingredients

4 tbsp almond flour
1 tbsp psyllium husk
Sea salt
Herbs to taste
2 tbsp EVOO

Method

- Roll the almond flour and psyllium husk into a pancake as explained in an earlier recipe, add the sea salt and herbs and brush with EVOO. Cut this base into triangles.
- Preheat the oven to 180°C. Arrange the triangles on an aluminium foil on the oven rack and bake for 10 minutes at 180°C.
- Reduce heat to 100°C and bake for another 10 minutes. Switch off the oven. Leave the triangles in the oven for 20 minutes. Keep an eye on them. If they get too brown, you can pull them out. Otherwise, leave them in to become crisp.
- Serve with any dip or chutney.

93. Roasted potatoes

Ingredients

½ kg baby red potatoes, parboiled

2 tbsp EVOO
2 cloves garlic
Italian seasoning
Salt and pepper to taste

Method

- Parboil baby potatoes with skin in a pan. Keep checking that they do not become too tender. Run them under cold water so that they become firm. Then slice the potatoes.
- Make a mix of EVOO, garlic and seasoning, and coat the potatoes. Arrange the potatoes with the cut sides down on a baking tray lined with baking paper.
- Roast at 200°C for 45–55 minutes, tossing every 15 minutes.

94. Quinoa tikki

Ingredients

1 cup quinoa
1 tbsp rice bran oil
1 big onion, chopped
1–2 green chillies, chopped (optional)
1 tbsp garlic paste
1 cup carrot, grated (optional)
½ cup fenugreek leaves, chopped
1 tsp chilli powder
½ tsp fresh cumin seeds
Salt to taste

Method

- Boil water in a pan, add a little salt and then the quinoa. Boil for 15–20 minutes and keep aside.
- Heat another pan, add rice bran oil, and add the onion, green chilli and garlic paste. Stir until the onion turns translucent.
- Add the carrot and fry for 3–4 minutes.
- Add the fenugreek leaves. Stir till all the water evaporates.
- Add chilli powder, cumin powder, salt and the boiled quinoa to this mixture. After 2 minutes, switch off the heat and leave aside to cool.
- When the mixture cools, shape into patties and put it in an air fryer at 180°C at level 5 or till crispy.
- Serve with chutney.

95. Falafel

Ingredients

2 cups amaranth flour seeds
1½ cup fresh coriander leaves
½ cup fresh dill, stems removed
1 small onion, quartered
7–8 garlic cloves, peeled
3–4 pieces black peppercorns
½ tbsp cumin seeds
6–7 coriander seeds
2 tbsp toasted sesame seeds
½ tsp baking powder

Salt to taste
Oil for frying

Method

- Fill a large bowl with water. Add the amaranth seeds and baking soda. The water should cover the amaranth seeds by at least 2 inches. Soak for 18 hours (longer if the amaranth seeds are still hard). When ready, drain the amaranth seeds and pat dry.
- Blend the amaranth seeds, coriander, dill, onion, garlic and spices till they form a coarse paste. Transfer to a container and cover tightly. Refrigerate for at least 1 hour or overnight.
- Add sesame seeds and baking powder. Shape the coarse mixture into ½-inch-thick balls. It helps to wet your hands before you do this.
- Add 3 inches of oil to a medium-sized saucepan and heat on medium heat until it bubbles. Carefully drop the falafel balls in the oil and fry for about 3–5 minutes till crispy. Fry in batches to not overcrowd the pan. Serve hot.

Note: You can also use bajra or buckwheat groats instead of amaranth seeds.

96. Sesame granola/chikki

Ingredients

100 gm white sesame seeds
150 gm organic jaggery powder

Method

- Spread a parchment sheet on a tray.

- Dry-roast the sesame seeds in a nonstick or heavy-bottomed pan on medium heat. Keep stirring continuously. In 6–7 minutes, the seeds will start crackling and change colour to light brown, giving off a roasted aroma.
- Lower the heat and add the jaggery powder while stirring. The jaggery will melt and coat the sesame seeds. You can add a spoon of water if it's too hard and difficult to stir. Mix for a minute and then pour it over the parchment sheet on the tray.
- Cover it with another parchment sheet and flatten it with the help of a rolling pin. All this has to be done very quickly because it sets immediately.
- Next, remove the sheets, break it into small pieces.

97. Dates squares

Ingredients

1 tsp olive oil
1 cup dates
1 tbsp almonds
1 tbsp pistachios
1 tbsp walnuts
2 tbsp poppy seeds

Method

- Heat oil in a pan and add the dates. Cook on low heat while stirring for 5–8 minutes or till it turns into a soft lump. Remove from heat and add the nuts.
- Flatten with a spatula, coat with poppy seeds and refrigerate to set. Cut into squares and store in an airtight container.

98. Quinoa cake

Ingredients

1 cup quinoa
3 cups water
2–3 apples
2 pinches of clove powder
A pinch of cinnamon powder
1 tsp sesame seeds

Method

- Cook the quinoa in 3 cups of water and allow it to cool.
- Peel and dice the apples and put them in a pan with 30 ml water and the clove and cinnamon powders. You can increase the cinnamon as per taste. Simmer for a minute and then reduce the heat. Cover the pan and cook for 7–8 minutes or till the apples are soft. Take off the heat but keep covered. Set aside for 30 minutes.
- Preheat the oven for five minutes at 200°C.
- Blend the cooled quinoa and apple mixture. Sprinkle sesame seeds and bake in the oven for 10 minutes at 200°C. If you want it crispier or harder, you can increase the time. Otherwise, allow it to cool for 40 minutes and then take the tray out of the oven.
- Serve as a snack with green tea.

99. Almond flour brownies

Ingredients

1⅓ cups almond flour

¼ cup rice flour
½ cup unsweetened cocoa powder
½ tsp baking soda
¼ tsp cinnamon (optional)
½ tsp sea salt
½ cup unsweetened applesauce
½ cup dates syrup (see p. 210)
⅓ cup unsalted almond butter
2 tsp natural vanilla extract (optional)
½ cup dairy-free semi-sweet chocolate chips

Method

- Preheat oven to 200°C.
- In a bowl, mix almond flour, rice flour, cocoa powder, baking soda, cinnamon and sea salt.
- Separately, blend applesauce, dates syrup, almond butter and vanilla extract in a blender till velvety.
- Combine both into a batter and add the chocolate chips.
- Line a baking pan with parchment paper. Spread the thick batter on the baking pan, and sprinkle more chocolate chips. Bake for 30 minutes. Leave in the oven for another 10 minutes. Take out and allow to cool for 1 hour at least. Then slice.
- The brownies will stay at room temperature for a day or two and in the refrigerator for up to 5 days. Almond flour brownies can be frozen too.

100. Vegan dark chocolate chip cookies

Ingredients

50 gm quinoa flour
50 gm white rice flour
½ cup almond butter
2 tbsp dates syrup (see p. 210)
2 tsp pure vanilla extract
¼ cup almond milk
1 tsp baking soda
¼ tsp salt
1 cup vegan dark chocolate chips

Method

- Mix the quinoa and rice flour well and keep aside.
- Preheat the oven to 200°C.
- Line baking pan with parchment paper.
- Using a handheld mixer, beat the almond butter and dates syrup together until creamy for about 2 minutes. Stir in the vanilla extract and almond milk slowly. Sprinkle the baking soda and salt on top of the flour. Mix on low speed until combined.
- Mix the chocolate chips into the dough.
- Use a scoop to take 1–2 tablespoons of dough for each ball; roll all the dough into balls and place on the prepared baking sheets about 2 inches apart. Bake for 9–12 minutes, until

golden-brown on the edges. They will appear soft at first but will firm up as they cool. Sprinkle with salt if desired.
- Let the cookies cool for 5 minutes, then remove from the oven to cool completely.

GRATITUDE

Without the people mentioned here, this book would still be stuck in my soul and never be in print.

- All my warrior patients who taught me repeatedly that each time we nourish and nurture, we heal.
- Prachi, Farah and Rohit, for your rock-solid faith in me.
- Aradhna, for being my strength, my fellow warrior healer with the miracle touch, my daughter, my bae.
- Vikram, for being my unconditional safe space to love and be loved.
- Anavi Bhushan Nugyal, for the quick and thoughtful design graphics.

NOTES

Scan this QR code to access the detailed notes.

NOTES

Scan this QR code to access the detailed notes.

FURTHER READING

RA Research and Therapy

https://arthritis-research.biomedcentral.com/articles/10.1186/ar2951

https://pubmed.ncbi.nlm.nih.gov/10451062/

Washington University School of Medicine. "Mind-body connection is built into brain." ScienceDaily. ScienceDaily, 19 April 2023. www.sciencedaily.com/releases/2023/04/230419125052.htm

Alternate nostril breathing: a systematic review of clinical trials International Journal of Research in Medical Sciences

https://www.msjonline.org/index.php/ijrms/article/view/3581#:~:text=Most%20of%20the%20studies%20included,autonomic%20nervous%20and%20cardiopulmonary%20systems

https://www.nhs.uk/conditions/rheumatoid-arthritis/diagnosis/

The cumulative long-term effects of sleep loss and sleep disorders have been associated with a wide range of deleterious health consequences including an increased risk of hypertension, diabetes, obesity, depression, heart attack, and stroke.

https://www.ncbi.nlm.nih.gov/books/NBK19961/# :~:text=The%20cumulative%20long%2Dterm%20effects,%2C%20heart%20attack%2C%20and%20stroke.

B-cell mediated disease: British Society of Immunology

https://www.immunology.org/public-information/bitesized-immunology/immune-dysfunction/b-cell-mediated-disease#:~:text=Autoimmunity,systemic%20lupus%20erythematosus%20(SLE).

Mayo Clinic

https://www.mayoclinic.org/diseases-conditions/addisons-disease/symptoms-causes/syc-20350293#:~:text=Primary%20adrenal%20insufficiency,which%20the%20body%20attacks%20itself.

Stress as a trigger of autoimmune disease

University Medical Center, Belgrade University, Serbia

https://pubmed.ncbi.nlm.nih.gov/18190880/#:~:text=It%20is%20presumed%20that%20the,altering%20or%20amplifying%20cytokine%20production.

https://www.emjreviews.com/allergy-immunology/article/genetically-modified-wheat-wheat-intolerance-and-food-safety-concerns/

ABOUT THE AUTHOR

Walks by the sea. Long asana holds. Deep breathing. Binge-watching comedy series and medical dramas. Treating mental health, autoimmune and cancer patients around the world. These are some of the things that keep Rachna Chhachhi engaged. After rheumatoid arthritis ravaged her life in 2006, she first healed herself and then dedicated her life to healing others like her. Rachna runs a registered non-profit, Kindness Practice Foundation, which creates awareness via camps, events and projects on nutrition, mental health and sustainability. Under the foundation, she runs a global support group for autoimmune warriors called The Autoimmune Community®.

Rachna has won many awards and hosts the largest non-profit annual awards platform for mental health and sustainability—The Restore Awards®, endorsed by the United Nations. A TEDx speaker and frequently on the jury of business magazines and forums to promote the next generation of well-being entrepreneurs, Rachna volunteers with cancer foundations and is regularly invited as a speaker at medical conferences to share her clinical papers on autoimmune diseases and cancer.

'RachnaRestores' was a nickname given to her by her healed patients and followers, which became her identity. Her website and social media handles are by the same name. She instituted the RachnaRestores Protocol®, which has healed thousands of patients across the world who had lost hope. The best description of her treatment methodology is: 'Heal from whatever they say you can't.'

This is Rachna's fifth book.

Follow Rachna on Instagram, Facebook, Twitter and YouTube via her handle RachnaRestores. Get in touch via email: healme@rachnarestores.com

HarperCollins *Publishers* India

At HarperCollins India, we believe in telling the best stories and finding the widest readership for our books in every format possible. We started publishing in 1992; a great deal has changed since then, but what has remained constant is the passion with which our authors write their books, the love with which readers receive them, and the sheer joy and excitement that we as publishers feel in being a part of the publishing process.

Over the years, we've had the pleasure of publishing some of the finest writing from the subcontinent and around the world, including several award-winning titles and some of the biggest bestsellers in India's publishing history. But nothing has meant more to us than the fact that millions of people have read the books we published, and that somewhere, a book of ours might have made a difference.

As we look to the future, we go back to that one word—a word which has been a driving force for us all these years.

Read.

     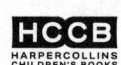